Nobody Knows
The Calories
I've Seen

Nobody Knows The Calories I've Seen

Arthur Sturges
Creator of "New Menu Cuisine"

M. EVANS & COMPANY, INC. NEW YORK

Library of Congress Cataloging-in-Publications Data

Sturges, Arthur.
    Nobody knows the calories I've seen / Arthur Sturges.
        p. cm.
    ISBM 0-87131-699-4 : $12.95
    1. Cookery. 2. Nutrition. I. Title.
TX714.S79   1992
641.5'63—dc20   92-13686

                                                                       CIP

M. Evans and Company, Inc.
216 East 49th Street
New York, New York 10017

Manufactured in the United States of America

9 8 7 6 5 4 3 2 1

DEDICATION

To Ellen, my wife, and best friend, I dedicate this book. For your hours and hours of typing and for your patience for the past 15 years. I can't make it without you.

A mention to my Mother, Penelope, whose persistence forced me to find a better way. Thanks Mom, for saving my life.

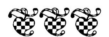

TABLE OF CONTENTS

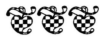

Introduction

We are killing ourselves. Men, women and children are unknowingly participating in a class action suicide that is slowly shortening their lives. A glitzy glut of misinformation from the media has suckered our society into believing it's the healthiest generation of Americans ever.

What we really are — is wrong. Americans are grossly overweight, unhealthy and uninformed. We have surpassed couch potato status and become rooted to the furniture and the t.v. We are nutritionally naive victims of multi-million dollar industries made up of food manufacturers, advertisers and health care companies. Their scheme is to convince consumers they're getting accurate and helpful information on food labels; information that implies these products are healthy, lower in fat, lower in sugar and higher in nutrition. And since most of us can't identify or even pronounce these ingredients, we're fat fools surviving on the typically American diet of misinformation covered in a glaze of exaggeration with just a dash of truth.

Some reports you see or read are correct and encouraging. Spa memberships are up while calorie intake is down, and maybe you look better as a result. But if you don't correctly understand what you're doing to the inside of your body, your outside won't matter. You'll still need a mortician to fix your face.

If you've been trying to learn more about what you eat by reading food label literature, stick to Shakespeare. It's easier. I'm a chef for goodness sake and I can't pronounce the ingredients listed. Nor can I tell you their functions.

In spite of ourselves, we suffer societal ignorance about the foods we eat and how they affect our health and weight. The one thing we do know is that proper nutrition has become confusing. And we don't need an expert to tell us that.

I learned all this from a cheesecake. When I realized how bad I felt after indulging in the creamy dessert, it finally dawned on me that I had to make some serious changes before I dropped dead earlier than I had intended.

I didn't become en"lite"ened overnight. I was in the restaurant business for a long time and I'm pretty good with food. After all, I've been eating it all my life. But I was too good for my own good, and not very happy about how I felt or how I looked. I began to think about change. I dreamed of one day wearing "One Size Fits All."

Once I accepted the fact that I needed to change virtually all of my behaviors, I became a "Born Again Chef," of sorts. I sold my restaurant and created new ways to prepare the same foods I loved. I call this "New Menu Cuisine."

As I started losing weight and feeling better about myself, I realized that the bigger success was that I had taken control of my weight concern. I learned to outsmart food manufacturers, advertisers and the diet "experts."

Since then, I have made it my crusade to teach you not to believe everything you read and hear, but to question. My mission is to save your life and the lives of your children, the next generation.

It's time we realize that we are killing our children as well as ourselves. America's youths have become addicted to junk food. They are what I call, "Junk Foodies." We must teach them and make them aware of the healthier way of living.

By traditional standards, I'm no expert; what I've become is what I call a "Foodtritionist," a combination dietician and nutritionist. A foodtritionist subscribes to the theory that through moderation and a basic understanding of the concepts regarding proper nutrition, you can enjoy eating, lose weight and get healthy. Sprinkle in exercise and you have a recipe for a great life.

I am thriving testimony of this theory's success. I have spent the greater portion of my 49 years battling my weight problem and the atrocious eating habits I acquired as a child. After seeing the "lite," I underwent a major metamorphosis and shed old habits as well as pounds. I still eat great meals, but now I feel well. I even enjoy exercise, which is the biggest change of all. I'm still heavy and still losing weight, but I'm healthy and happy.

Maybe you think you're achieving success and good health because you take time to read food labels instead of trashy novels and you've worked up a sweat trying to figure out how many grams of fat make cellulite. But admit it, you don't know what those multisyllabic words called ingredients mean? When something says 7 grams of fat, that doesn't tell you anything significant either.

There's a better way. Follow my simple rule—Fat is Fat. Fat Makes Fat. No matter where it comes from be it animal, vegetable or mineral, fat will put more fat on you. The less fat you consume, the easier it will be for your body to burn up what you've been lugging around and plugging into your arteries all these years. But to reduce fat, you have to be able to identify it on those labels. Helping you do that is part of my mission.

When a canned pasta product loaded with beef and cheese is hyped as being 95 percent fat free, and we accept that without question, we become fatheads. Beef and cheese have fat. There's no getting around it. When you use "lite" oil, the term "lite" only refers to the color. Oil is fat. And your body can't take it.

Do you see how misleading and confusing this stuff is? Do you understand why this information is so important?

If you need a visual aid, remove the skin of a chicken and try to destroy it in the garbage disposal. You can't. If you can't wreck it up with a machine, why would you think your body could get rid of it?

Fat is a big problem in our society and it's really reached a crisis point, just like it did in my life. As a nation we spend a fortune on medical research to prevent our hearts from attacking us, to relieve our high-pressured blood and to let our livers live longer. Yet, we ignore researchers' findings and continue to eat and behave in dangerous ways, daring our bodies to react.

It's safe to say we all want to live longer. But in many cases, you can't have what you want unless you work for it.

You've heard all this before, but sometimes it takes a stronger message to make the point so think about this. Heart attacks may be the leading cause of death in this country, but just because you have one doesn't mean you'll leave this world so quick. You owe that possibility to all that medical research you've been financing over the years. If your heart just beats you up a bit and leaves you to live, think about how your life will change.

7

First of all, you will endure unimaginable pain and fright during and after the attack itself. The initial attack is followed by an ambulance ride, which on its own is stressful enough to cause one's ticker to panic. You'll probably go from the emergency room to an Intensive Care Unit, where no one can visit you for very long (you can't even receive flowers), followed by a lengthy recovery, which means missing work. You will undergo a complete overhaul of your lifestyle, which you should have done in the first place to avoid the aforementioned scenario.

There's more. Are you sure you're insured? Can you cover your recovery? And did it occur to you that your family will not enjoy the emotional adventure they will experience throughout your ordeal?

Meanwhile, your kids are consuming all kinds of stuff at school as well as at home. They aren't immune from heart failure, diabetes or even gallstones thanks to their early start on body trashing. The garbage they eat from vending machines at school, in front of the t.v. and at the "playground" (also known as The Mall) is greasing up their insides, prepping their bodies for a parade of problems. Most of today's youngsters can't even pass the President's Council on Physical Fitness tests anymore. Youngsters smoke earlier and more than any other generation. Face it, your children are dying.

And focusing on the bigger picture, these same youngsters who are fueling themselves with fats, will someday be leading our nation, our states, cities, schools, museums etc. Will they have enough confidence in themselves and the good health needed to take over the world's future?

Now, are you catching my drift? It's a much bigger issue than one of losing a few pounds and looking good. It's a matter of wanting to stay alive and well for a long time.

I know of what I speak. Like the title of this book, nobody knows the calories I've seen or the number of experts I've visited. In fact, I've seen more experts than calories and they've had as many different degrees of interest as there are degrees on my oven.

I once asked a dietician for an eating plan based on calorie intake and the first question she asked was, "What foods do you like?" I hesitated and answered meekly, "I like hot dogs." Feeling more secure after verbalizing my fondness

8

for frankfurters, I exhibited a bit more confidence and added, "In fact, I love hot dogs."

Why wouldn't anyone love hot dogs, I thought to myself. They're nothing but salt and fat—the basics of All-American ethnic food. (Baseball legend Babe Ruth ate dog after dog to the point where he became ill.)

Her response was, "Well if you like hot dogs I suppose we can fit them into your diet." Translation: "Scale back on the weenies, fella." The point is, she should have, but never said no, despite knowing that hot dogs just aren't any good for anyone.

It doesn't take an expert to know that too much fat significantly contributes to serious health problems and early death. I'm not saying a carrot cuisine is the answer either. Look at the picture of me on the cover of this book. Do I look like I live on alfalfa sprouts? No. But I do look happy. When you read this book and try my "New Menu Cuisine" creations, you'll understand how my philosophy destroys the "Triple D Theory" of diets, denial and disappointment.

I believe that if "bad" foods are consumed in moderation, almost anything you like can be enjoyed without guilt or gain. And here's how you do it. Figure you eat 21 meals a week. Of that total, 18 or 19 or those can be low-fat, healthy menus. The others can be anything you want, in moderation of course. If you stick to this routine, your cravings for sweets and fats will change for the better. Begin to exercise, too, and you'll lose weight. You will start feeling better physically and emotionally.

It's taken me almost a half century to figure all this out and the hard way I might add. Now I want to expose the hype and show you how to focus on the information you really need, but aren't getting or don't understand. I want you to develop a simple, but accurate understanding of calories, fats and cholesterol and how they relate to your good health and staying alive. You don't need to "diet" to eat smarter. You just need to make a choice: life or death.

Let's not diet, let's do it.

Did I Eat That?
(D.I.E.T.)

It ain't over til the fat lady sings, but if she doesn't start worrying about what she eats, she won't even hum. We all have to worry about what and how we eat or we'll have to form a chubby chorus and belt out the fat folk blues.

The Battle of the Bulge has become a war of wits as experts and uneducated victims of weight and poor nutrition problems duke it out over who has the best recipe for weight loss. And throughout this conflict, we have turned into gluttons for expert advice. Unfortunately, much of what we hear is more complex than the best carbohydrates.

To me, understanding the basics of nutrition, factually but simply, is the best way to make a point successfully. It's this philosophy that has attracted my audience and kept everyone informed with minimal damage to their egos and maximum success in finding good health.

The premise of this book is based on my philosophy — weight loss and good health bolstered by a healthy dose of self-confidence — can be acquired through common sense, dedication and discipline. Speaking as someone who continues to fight a lifelong weight problem, I have an astute understanding of what's involved in overhauling a grossly unhealthy lifestyle that survived on too much of all the wrong things. It took fortysomething years of no success for me to learn that I could lose weight and get healthy and enjoy myself at the same time; and all without a lot of hooey from the experts.

The root of my philosophy is that "Fat Makes Fat." Now, is that easy or what? The more fat you ingest the more you will lug in your gut, your arteries and in your head. Our bodies simply don't metabolize fats the way proteins and carbohydrates are burned up by this great machine we call human.

We all know to count the calories we consume. But it's not the number of calories, but the type of calories we must worry about.

Do you know what a calorie is? Do you need to know? Yes. (It doesn't get that simple.) Without drowning in physics, let's just understand that a calorie is the unit of energy that makes our bodies work. Calories, like car fuel, burn up. When you consume more calories than you burn up, you gain weight. You get unhappy. And if most of your calorie intake comes from fats, you're in the deep weeds and sinking fast. We must learn to get the bulk of our calories from more efficient sources such as proteins and carbohydrates, which burn up easier. Of course, there are problems in these areas, too, but we'll get to that.

The American Heart Association recommends we limit our daily fat intake to 30 percent of our total intake. However, we Americans actually consume almost 20 percent more, which means about half our intake is fats.

Saturated, unsaturated, monounsaturated or polyunsaturated-fat is fat. And the problem with fats is that they stay in your system, grabbing hold in obvious and not so obvious locations, including your arteries, creating an obstruction thicker than the Berlin Wall. Cosmetically, you discover your thighs have become lumpy, your rear end takes longer following you into a room and you no longer can see your loafers loaf.

Even more serious, however, is that some fats, specifically those from animals, contain cholesterol which contributes to plugging arteries while clearing the way for serious heart problems. Fats from other sources may not contain killer cholesterol, but they have the ability to harden and aggravate existing cholesterol levels in your system. Either way, you won't be going to the movies anymore if you continue to invite fats and other poisons to enter your body. So let's develop a simple understanding of where we can make changes.

CHOLESTEROL

I could devote this entire book to cholesterol, but it's too much techno-trition for our purposes. Cholesterol is not like Dow Jones — it's not supposed to go up and down. I want to keep this simple but accurate so here's an overview of how this substance affects us.

Picture a cross section of pipe that started out crystal clean and over time developed a substantial buildup of minerals. The original hole became significantly smaller due to this buildup, drastically restricting any flow. The same happens in the arterial passages when cholesterol builds up. Get the picture?

The way to overcome this is to know what foods contain cholesterol and then to not eat them. You wouldn't swallow rat poison would you? It's the same thing.

Remember our basic premise "Fat Makes Fat." Add this to your memory: "Cholesterol Comes From Animals." For example, eggs come from chickens. That means cholesterol. Butter comes from cream, which comes from, yes, another animal; the cow. It's so easy, so important, yet it has gotten so confusing.

There's an abundance of books detailing the facts about cholesterol, but simply stated, stay away from saturated fats and opt for polyunsaturated and use them minimally. (I will show you how in my recipe section and you'll be able to see how easy it is to make a change in the way you cook.)

Meanwhile, we also must be aware of the existence of tropical oils in many of the products we consume. Tropical oils aren't healthy and as that fact has been made more public, more food manufacturers are finding alternatives in their production. However, some aren't and you must teach yourself to investigate those food labels and know which ingredients are the ones to avoid.

Tropical oils are taboo because of their ability to congeal or harden once in your system and raise blood cholesterol drastically. They are easy to recognize because of where they originate. For example, coconut oils and palm oils both hail from plant life found in tropical climates.

It is the result of these oils or fats that plug up arterial paths, creating the potential for great heartache—literally.

So what do you do? Learn to read; you must become label literate. By doing so you will be able to determine the good and bad ingredients in the foods you buy and prepare. Stick to the polyunsaturated fats, using them with restraint.

Along with learning what's in a product you should and can learn how to understand the quantities that are listed. You can become a Fat Detective (although you don't want to be a fat anything). The following is a simple calculation that will provide you with an accurate measurement of just how much fat that product really contains. I stress the accuracy of this formula because often times, food labels that boast reduced or low fat contents are misleading and it takes a bit of math and initiative to get around this misinformation. Warning: be leery of a product that doesn't advertise its nutritional information. Just like we dress to cover our less attractive parts, so do food manufacturers. Odds are, the product is fantastically high in fat and swimming in sodium.

Here's your mathematic mode to discovery. Fat contains nine, count 'em, nine calories per gram. Multiply this number by the number of grams listed. For example: A jar of mayonnaise lists a serving size as one tablespoon with 100 calories per serving. The label also lists the fat content as 11 grams.

According to our fat finding formula, we take the number of grams of fat and multiply by nine; that sum is divided by the number of calories per serving, which gives you an accurate percentage of fat content. Here's math in action:

Multiply the 11 grams from the mayonnaise by nine which gives us 99. Divide that 100 calorie serving into 99. The answer is 99. In plain English, that means 99 percent or the majority of calories in this product come from fat. See how tricky, how misleading labels can be? See how easy and scary discovering the truth can be?

$$\frac{\text{Grams of Fat X 9}}{\text{Total Calories per Serving}} = \text{of Fat Calories in Food}$$

Later, I will give you some tips on reducing the fat content while still using mayonnaise as well as some other simple methods to remove fat from your favorite foods without destroying their flavor. But first, there are still a couple of issues we must address before we get to the fun stuff.

SALT

You may be the salt of the earth to your friends, but you could end up becoming part of the earth if you overdose on salt. Like cholesterol, too much is too bad.

Call it sodium or salt, it's the same chemical compound and it causes hypertension. Some salt users are able to retain water better than the mightiest camel.

Salt consumption is serious business. The resulting reservoir inside your body because of salt, causes pressure to build up creating the condition — High Blood Pressure, aka Hypertension.

Just like fat and cholesterol, you don't need this stuff and you can cut back with the greatest of ease. Salt is an acquired taste and one you can lose in a few months by cutting it from cooking and stopping haphazard shaking it over your meal before you've even tasted your food. As a start, I suggest taping over all the salt shaker holes except two.

If you can't quit cold turkey, at least restrict yourself to minimum mealtime use only. At least you'll have a bit of control over how much you use. Cutting back slowly is better than not at all.

FIBER

Nature's Broom is a more attractive term for describing the role fiber plays in our system. The fiber factor has become as confusing as anything else connected with today's nutrition industry so here's another of my easy to understand explanations.

Fiber is the stuff that sweeps out the byproducts the body doesn't use. While fiber keeps our process of elimination steady, the medical community in recent years has stressed fiber's importance in possible cancer prevention.

You can't see fiber, but it's fairly easy to find and especially in natural foods such as fruits, vegetables and grains, some of which work better than others. Beans are a superior source of fiber as are potatoes, broccoli, and even strawberries.

We've also heard a lot about bran, another excellent source for fiber. And the easiest ways to find bran fiber is in breakfast cereals, muffins and breads containing bran. Many cereals are advertised based on the fiber benefit. It's best to get fiber naturally than through artificial methods such as laxatives. And changing to a more healthy, nutritious diet can accomplish an improved fiber intake.

Although fiber is necessary to keep your digestion system (specifically your bowels) on track, like anything else, too much of a good thing can become a problem. An over-dose of fiber can block you up just as badly as if you didn't have any fiber, so don't go crazy with it. We really need just enough to keep our systems running smoothly and regularly. The recommended level is 25 to 40 grams daily.

Additionally, fiber performs another function. Most high fiber products are low in calories and low in or free of fat. However, fibrous products create a feeling of fullness and help us eat less even when we don't know it.

PROTEINS

Proteins are the elements we use to fuel our bodies. They provide us with amino acids which help in the growth and repair of our cells. Proteins are vital to our existence, but there are good sources and some not so good. And, as usual, the not so good sources can be deadly. Everyone knows there is a lot of protein in meats like beef, but there's also a huge amount of fat. Our need for protein doesn't justify eating what I like to call a big "old cowboy steak" or chewing enough cheese to choke a mouse. Both are high fat sources and more harmful than healthy.

Strong protein alternatives include lean vegetables (which by now you've seen can do no wrong), grains, yogurt and skim milk to name a few. Meats are alright, but they must be lean cuts (a 3-4 oz portion only; not a 16 oz. steak) or poultry, fish or pork. The same goes for beef.

CARBOHYDRATES

Carbohydrates energize us and keep us feeling full of spark. Unlike the short-lived energy boost we get from sugar in candy or elsewhere, carbohydrates have proven to be a steady source of strong support. This is exemplified by athletes, who increase their carbohydrate intake before they compete so they are able to participate at their maximum capabilities.

Simple carbohydrates are sugar. In their natural state, such as skim milk or fruit, they are acceptable. Once refined, sugar is sugar and it is high in calories and low in vitamins and nutrients. Use sparingly.

Complex carbohydrates are somewhat lower in fat and calories. They contain good amounts of vitamins and minerals. They are found in beans, potatoes, grains and breads (and I don't mean that soft stuff we know as white bread). I'm talking hearty and healthy whole grain breads and pastas. Yes, you can have spaghetti. (Just go easy on the sauce and cheese. And follow my recipe later in the book.)

Carbohydrates are easy to keep handy, easy to prepare and easy to digest. They play an important role in healthy nutrition and overall good health. So enjoy.

Good nutrition boils down to this: fats, proteins and carbohydrates. Remember, proteins make us strong and healthy, carbohydrates keep us going while fats hang on us.

The key to understanding all of this is the desire to be healthy and thus, happy. It's a complete process of changing eating habits, starting a regular exercise routine and sticking with it, and even changing your vocabulary. If you adopt my theories and my way of living, you will cut calories, fats and the word "diet." It's a negative and later we'll talk about cutting out those, too. The first three letters in this word spell doom so don't use it anymore unless as an acronym for "Did I Eat That?"

2

I Shop, Therefore I Eat

All of this advice and information looks great on paper, doesn't it? My goal is for you to look great and feel great. It's putting it into action that will really make you a believer. And one important thing to learn is to make educated decisions. And that means you have to outsmart the advertisers when you shop for your groceries.

Okay, so you can occasionally munch a handful of M&M's or a scoop of ice cream. But they shouldn't be included on your grocery shopping list. And if they're not on your list, then some of those foods you want to scale back on shouldn't mysteriously make their way into your shopping wagon either.

The best way to accomplish this method is to shop for groceries according to a plan. First you must try to not breach the ultimate taboo; food shopping when you're hungry.

You remember doing that in your lifetime, don't you? Sure; you brought home canned tamales, two chocolate cakes from the store bakery, cream cheese for your bagels and three varieties of potato chips.

This is costly in more ways than one and something I realized while unloading several empty Twinkie boxes and candy containers as I was going through the checkout line. At least I paid for what I ate.

You must shop with a plan. You've got to know what you need before you go and then stick to buying only those items listed. There's no need to stroll for sweet rolls or browse for brownies. Even though I can smell the bakery from the parking lot, I force myself to avoid it.

Grocery shopping can soothe the soul, break the wallet and fill the refrigerator. But like everything else in this life-style change, we must correct the shopping habits that have carried us forward into the battle of the bulge. Envision the grocery store now as a testing ground for your newfound label literacy as well as your will to succeed.

Remember, you're not only battling the bulge but the boys from Madison Avenue who have created packaging and advertising concepts that convince you to buy their products. Who cares whether they're good for you? You do, that's why you're reading this book.

In addition to the information I've provided about ingredients and fat content calculation, don't be afraid to apply common sense, the best deciding factor of all. For example, when a canned pasta product contains red meat and carries a label that boasts fat free, or even low-fat, think again. How can that be? It can't. That's when you use the other data you've learned.

The same can be said when margarine or biscuit mix is advertised as cholesterol free. That only means animal fats weren't used. Odds are, the product still contains a lot of fat and you know what that means. You simply must know what you are eating and that means you must know what you're buying.

Dairy products, for instance, present questions, confusion and unhappiness. All those different kinds and different percentages; what do they mean and which is best? As you shiver past the dairy case, remember — don't use anything but low-fat yogurt, very low fat cottage cheese. There now is also non-fat yogurt and cottage, ricotta and mozarella cheeses on shelves. And while the variety of milks may be enticing (along with the packaging) there isn't enough difference in them to make a difference in you so your best bet is skim milk. The fat has been skimmed off. Again, easy. No confusion here. Another example of common sense — avoid heavy cream.

What isn't commonly known is that dairy substitutes aren't the best alternatives to cream. These products may be low in calories, but about 90 percent of their caloric count comes from fats. (You can test this with the fat finding calculation.) Mind boggling, isn't it? Stick to skim milk to muddy up your occasional coffee.

There also is the issue of cheese, lots and lots of cheese. Cheese is very high in fat and cholesterol, which you should already have figured. So the smartest thing is to avoid it. But there is Sap Sago. Grated it smells like old sneakers, but it's pretty good on pasta instead of Parmesan or Romano.

The meats section, too, is a tough area. You'll know you shopped on an empty stomach when you get home and discover you purchased heavily marbled beef. That's the tastiest, but unhealthiest kind. It's prime trouble.

If you must eat meat, choose lean ones, the tough ones. In my recipes, you'll learn how to cook and enjoy it.

And while you're not buying fatty meats, don't buy internal organ meat, as well. Liver and kidney contain soaring cholesterol levels that could launch your heart into "obit." Pork is good meat, but only use tenderloin because it's very lean.

Obviously we don't live by bread alone, but there are some available that are so tasty and nutritious they could serve as a single course. However, like all other foods, you have to be sure about the contents. You can and should determine the contents and nutritional value of breads and cereals, which are included on their labels. A lot of those low-cal breads are high in sugars, something that may enhance the flavor and your weight problem besides.

Beans are included in the breads and grains categories. As I mentioned earlier, they provide protein and complex carbohydrates — two very good things. But some people aren't keen on bean so you may have to acquire a taste. My recipes will help you there.

And don't forget about the fresh vegetables and fruits. Canned are okay, too, but many are packed in heavy syrup which contributes to you being heavy. However, if you can't find fresh, all you have to do is rinse off the canned versions in running water.

As you begin shopping for more fresh foods and healthier foods, you may also notice a decrease in your grocery bill. Those snack cakes, chips and candies are expensive! Without them, your grocery bill may enjoy a reduction as well.

A little bit of knowledge can be very dangerous or very beneficial and in our case, it's what will save our lives. Soon meal planning and food shopping according to the New Menu Cuisine will become routine.

Other healthy shopping tips are available from the American Heart Association. You can just call or write to learn more about what you can do to save your heart from ache.

And you may be more encouraged to do so when you start seeing some real changes not only in your own weight reduction, but your overall health and energy levels, as well as your pocketbook. As you get in the habit of buying more fresh vegetables and fruits, and eating more pastas and rice and less meat, your grocery bills should start to reduce along with your figure.

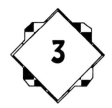

Fat Chance For Kids

When Junior was a little less than two years old he was quite the little pudge. Everyone said so. You always responded with the old wive's tale that a fat baby is a healthy baby.

Well, Junior is seven now and moves a little less than his playmates because he's still a bit round. It's baby fat, he'll lose it, is your answer?

Think again. Junior is headed for a lifelong weight problem compounded by the powerful potential for heart problems that currently affect so many American adults. It's time parents did something about these avoidable health problems. Speaking as someone who grew up overweight, I can't stress enough that you must teach your child how to eat healthy. If your child is young, there is no easier time to accomplish the deed at a time in your child's life when adopting a regimen of eating good foods is relatively easy to achieve. You're never to young to eat correctly. Healthy eating has no age limit.

Since educating your kids begins at home why not start with nutrition. In addition to training them not to talk to strangers and not to play in traffic, you can teach your kids not to eat foods that will eventually kill them. Your goal is to teach them to make good choices when they eat away from the home and away from you.

While parents live in fear their children will become drug addicts, we must also acknowledge that our children have become addicted to junk food or as I call them — "Junk Foodies."

Forget the fable that a fat baby is a healthy baby and that the extra pounds will magically disappear as the child gets older. And for goodness sake, don't feed your kids just to keep them quiet.

This is the kind of behavior that has created our new

generation of overweight and unhealthy youngsters and teens. With all the fat and fast food available to our children, it's no surprise that some children's cholesterol levels are outrageously high. Even some have scored with high cholesterol levels. The groundwork for our children's future is being laden with fat, empty calories and early death.

We are the adults. We are in charge. And we must save our children from an unnecessary and lifelong struggle with weight and poor health. It's not something with which to kid around.

4

Fat Man On A Bicycle

You say you can't move. You say you don't want to move. You're too tired. You don't have the time, the interest, the stamina. You swoon at the thought of sweating.

Well, too bad. If you want to lose weight, if you want to get healthy then you're going to have to steer away from the refrigerator and into an exercise program. It's the only way to lose weight and feel better physically and emotionally. There isn't a reduction program worth its salt that doesn't include working out in some form.

There was a point in my life where the only exercise I got was eating my meals quickly. That says it all, doesn't it? Maybe for you right now, the most exercise you get is trying to come up with new excuses why you can't work out. After a while, that gets to be more exhausting than just doing it. Think how much easier your life would be if you would get it over with.

I promise, once you start an exercise program you like, eventually you'll get as hooked as you were to your favorite dessert. Don't forget, exercise is one of the components that will allow you to continue having your favorite dessert on occasion.

This is no con. You will find that if you miss a workout, you really will miss it. When you find a routine you like, you can start out slowly, but as your stamina increases, it's likely your interest will increase as well. And you'll start to feel better quickly, too. You'll look better. You will be better.

There are as many options for exercise as there are fad diets. You may have to try a few before you find the one you like best.

Generally speaking, there are two different kinds of exercise, aerobic and anaerobic. Both are beneficial, but in different ways.

Aerobic exercise is what works your cardiovascular system, meaning your heart gets pumping. To be effective, aerobic workouts require your heart and lungs to function at a higher than normal rate and a constant pace for a specific time limit, such as 20 minutes. The goal is to get your system pumping hard enough to burn off fat, which is the benefit of aerobics.

Anaerobic exercise is more effective in improving muscle tone and strength. The cardiovascular system gets a less rugged workout and in short spurts rather than over an extended time period.

The overall benefits and ease of getting started with aerobics are what have made these kinds of exercises so popular. That's what all those video tapes advertised on television at 5 a.m. are all about.

Aerobic exercises don't mean you have to squeeze into shiny tights and swat at others stepping on you in an aerobic dance class. Bicycling, (my personal favorite), walking, running, jumping rope are all fantastic options that are easy to start, and don't cost a lot of money. Getting up from the couch to change the channel on the t.v. does not constitute aerobic exercise.

However, before you begin any exercise program, please see your doctor first so you know how to start safely and proceed without getting hurt. This is vital to your success.

Let's talk about what's available in the way of sweating our way to slenderhood. You see now that you have a lot of options. Let me offer you a few (I've tried almost all of them at some point). Despite the hype, you don't have to join a health club, you don't have to don fancy workout clothes or embarrass yourself. You can buy an exercise tape and begin a gentle workout in the privacy of your home and in your favorite sweats or whatever's comfortable. There's no one to bother you or to make you self-conscious.

These video workouts are available at different levels, ranging from beginner to advanced or high impact. You can start slow and see if you like it.

While it may seem strange and uncomfortable to huff and puff your way through a workout, keep in mind that that's the purpose of the routine. That's how you burn off fat.

If you want to huff and puff fresh air, there's always running, which is a tough route, and one that should be considered with caution and an understanding that it's strenuous right from the start. That may be why walking has attracted such an audience in recent years.

Walking with vigor requires the same amount of work from your heart and lungs, and burns off calories and fat just as running does. But it's easy and you already know how to do it. You've had years of training.

I suggest that you start by buying a good pair of walking shoes and stroll at least five minutes slowly, pick up the pace for about 20 to 25 minutes and wind up with a five-minute cool down. If that's too much, just go at your own comfortable pace until you feel up to increasing the pitter patter of your little feet.

And like the postman, rain, hail and sleet don't have to stop you from this routine. Treadmills are available virtually everywhere and at a range of prices.

Swimming also is an excellent choice, but you have to find a body of water in which to place your body. Swimming incorporates your entire body with a minimum of stress to any one area, unlike running, which can rub away your knees over time. Your cardiovascular system works at a constant pace and fat burns off and all is fine in the pool.

But my favorite exercise is bicycling. I've tried the others and this is what brings me great pleasure and success. Since I started I have lost 105 pounds. Each day my wife, Ellen, and I don shorts, our helmets and push those pedals around town. It's become a great way to start the day. We feel better, we handle stress better and because we've imbibed in all this exercise at the beginning of the day, we're less likely to blow our success by eating something filled with fat.

I should admit that I've really gotten hooked on this biking stuff. I buy old bikes and fix them up for friends. I persuade others to take up the sport and join us on long weekend outings through the countryside or through the downtown area. We stop for breakfast and continue on our way and it's all very social. See, exercise can be fun.

But believe me, it was no picnic getting started. The first day we rode, we pedaled all of five miles. I felt as if we had pedaled to the end of the earth. And there was another problem I hadn't expected. My rear end, my posterior, my gluteus maximus was hurting, seriously hurting. This sure wasn't how I remember my childhood days when a bike was my only means of transportation and when I rode miles and miles and miles.

Since then I've discovered gel seats, which soften the ride. My goal is to fit into "one-size-fits-all" biker pants, those spandex things with the built-in crotch pads.

Basically, what I'm saying is that before you invest in a bicycle, test ride different models at reputable bike shops. Don't invest in a chain store brand. And talk to knowledgeable salespeople. Ask to see the buyer's guide, which will help you make a better choice.

There are a lot of bikes to choose from, some with no gears, a few gears or a bunch of gears. Let the sales people help you determine what you are looking for according to how far and how often you intend to ride. The best thing about these exercise ideas is that you don't have to spend a fortune.

If you walk or run, invest in good socks and shoes. The first time I walked, after all of 15 minutes I thought I was going to drop in the street. I was pooped and I had a blister the size of a silver dollar on both heels. Don't let this happen to you.

If you take an aerobics class, again, buy some shoes. You don't want to get started with one of these activities and then get hurt. You can look as unathletic as you want and get yourself in shape. A wrecked up pair of shorts, torn t-shirts, or dirty shoes are acceptable. Just be sure you have the right equipment to participate safely.

I'm not saying it can't get costly. Some health club memberships cost staggering amounts of money and require you to sign up for more than one year. (There's always the local YMCA). Running shoes can cost more than $100. There are discount sporting goods stores all over the place, which will help you save some bucks.

Treadmills can run up into the thousands. Again, discount stores offer sturdy equipment and reduced rates. Sometimes the classified section of your local newspaper is a great resource for second-hand equipment. You have choices.

Getting fit won't and can't happen overnight. But you do feel improvements pretty quickly. As long as you stick with eating healthy and working out consistently, you'll feel your endurance increase, you'll feel stronger, sleeker and more fit.

But the most important piece of equipment you'll need is self-discipline. That's what makes exercise work.

And just for a little boost of encouragement, I've included two pages of illustrations to demonstrate some simple stretches that should be done before (and also after) any exercise routines. Warm up for at least 10 minutes prior to your exercise session and cool down for about 5 minutes after.

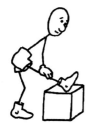

#1. HAMSTRING STRETCH

Put right heel on a step or chair and right hand on right thigh. With back straight, bend forward slightly at the waist, pressing down on thigh until you feel the stretch behind your knee and thigh. Hold 5 seconds and repeat with other leg.

#2. LEG FLEX

Sit on floor and extend legs forward about 18" apart. Slowly, point and flex right foot 8 times; then left foot 8 times. Then from your hip, slowly roll each leg inward and outward 8 times.

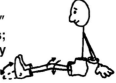

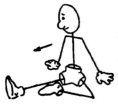

#3. HAMSTRING STRETCH #2

Sit on floor with right leg extended out front and left knee bent so foot is flat against inner right knee. With hands extended behind you for balance, gently lean forward to feel stretch. Come back up and repeat 3 times. Repeat with other leg.

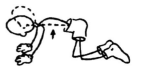

#4. CAT CURLS

Kneel on hands and knees (hands 18" apart and knees hip width apart). Keep chin tight to your chest, stomach tightened toward your spine and arch your back up like a cat. Gently return to flat position. Repeat 5 times.

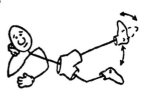

#5. LEG LIFTS

Lie on your side on floor, hand supporting head, other hand on floor in front of you for balance. Roll hips slightly forward placing weight on front arm. With bottom leg slightly back, top leg straightened and foot flexed, lift and lower foot 8 times. Now point top foot and raise and lower it 8 times. Repeat with other leg.

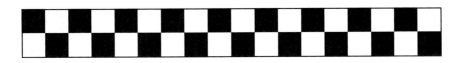

#6. INNER THIGH TIGHTENER

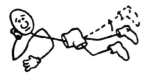

Lie on floor in same position as in Leg Lifts. With bottom leg straight and other leg slightly bent in front, point bottom foot and lift leg from the hip 10 times. When lowering foot, don't let it touch floor. Repeat with other leg on top.

#7. KNEE LIFTS

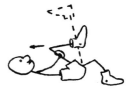

Lie on floor, on back, with knees bent and feet flat on floor. With both hands behind right thigh, pull bent leg to chest. Extend leg toward ceiling. Bend knee back to chest. Repeat 5 times and then repeat with other leg.

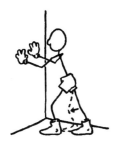

#8. ACHILLES AND CALF STRETCH

Facing a wall and with feet back 2 ft., place hands on wall at shoulder level. With straightened right leg extended slightly back, keeping foot flat on floor, bend left knee gently until you feel stretch in right leg. Hold 5 seconds and repeat with other leg.

#9. SHIN AND CALF STRETCH

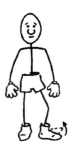

Stand straight with hand on wall to stabilize you. Lift left foot, flex and point and make circles with ankle. Repeat 6 times and repeat with other foot.

#10. 1/2 SIT-UPS

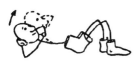

Lie on floor, on your back with hands under your head for support. With knees bent, feet flat on floor and pelvis pressing downward, lift shoulders off floor and back down. Repeat 10 times.

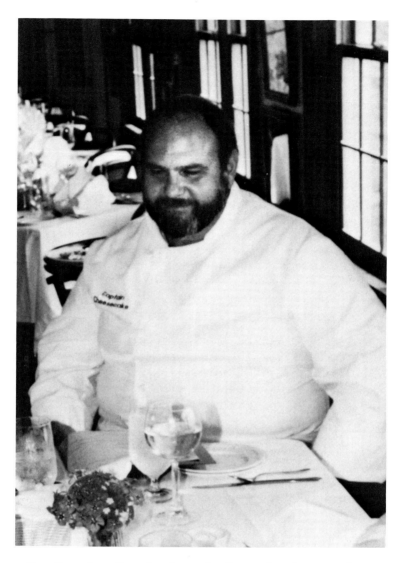

Here I am in unhappier days; the days when I was at least 100 pounds heavier and busy avoiding having my picture taken. Now that I'm slimmer, I love myself and the camera.

They Like Me, I Like Me

If I could just wear 32-inch waist slacks I'd be happy. If I could just eat all the cheesecake I wanted I'd be happy. If only I didn't have to worry about how much salt I use, I'd be happy.

Well, I can't do any of these things and guess what, I'm pretty darned happy. I wasn't always euphoric, but that's probably an accurate assessment of my personality today. I'm still heavy, but getting slimmer and more handsome every day. At least that's what I tell everyone. The point of all this is that my attitude is positive. Because of that I enjoy my life, my wife, my family and friends. I still want to lose more weight, but I'm not consumed by my goal. It does not control my life. I do.

I wasn't always this way, but it's how I plan to stay and it's how I plan to succeed in getting and staying healthy for the rest of my days. It's all up to me. The same applies to you.

We've talked about fixing our systems with the right foods and of getting rid of the poisons that plug our hearts. But in addition, we also need to stick to a healthy menu of self-esteem, a positive philosophy.

Getting healthy is more than just eating well and keeping off fat. It includes good emotional health as well. So if you lose a lot of weight but still don't see yourself in a positive way, you need to do more. You need to change your outlook and that means you must believe that you will achieve the results you want. You must learn to like yourself. But to do that you must set some tough priorities and doing that may be harder than trying to shed 10 pounds. Because of losing pounds, you may have to dump a job, an activity of a person, the someone who is a negative in your life.

I've devised a way to get started with this process of

getting rid of the negatives and inhaling the positive. Strip down to your birthday suit, stand on the scale and face the music, which actually means the mirror. If you're really serious about changing your life, you will step on that scale and accept the numbers. But accept them in a positive way. Don't take three digits and get down in the dumps. Apply a little emotional mathematics and turn those numbers into guidelines, and commit yourself to changing them to digits that are acceptable to you. Because you do know that it can be done.

Some experts recommend avoiding a daily weigh-in. I, however, prefer to check my weight daily so that I stay on course. If I don't like what I see one day, I'll set my mind to correct it. I see this as progress, I see this as taking control.

Sure, you'll go up and down on the scale occasionally. Yes, you'll hit plateaus and won't lose weight, but they are temporary. And, yes, sometimes you'll eat something you weren't supposed to have. So what. You won't do it again.

In the grand scheme of things, what's most important is that you believe in yourself and that you take control of your life and actually enjoy yourself during this process of change. You will find that by eating better, you naturally will begin to feel better physically, which in turn will help you feel better emotionally. One feeds off the other and that's what you're after.

This taking charge stuff is rewarding and is what boosts self-esteem. You will appreciate your new healthy behaviors and thus, it will dawn on you; you'll like yourself.

But you must adopt this method of positive thinking. It can be difficult, but you can commit yourself to change and by eating better you've already gotten started. The discipline of rejecting bad foods and sticking to an exercise program can teach you how to believe in yourself. For example, when I take friends bicycling with me and they comment on the distance I've ridden, I take pride in what they've noticed; how far I've taken myself. Of course, they think I'm beaming about the mileage I've pedaled, when I'm thinking about how I've changed my whole outlook on life.

It's not easy to do. But there's no point in putting it off either. You don't have to wait until January 1 or next Monday to change your life or your attitude. If it happens to be 3:30

in the afternoon and you're ready to make a change and start liking yourself, then do it, then and there. Try while you're reading this book. Don't you feel better about taking the time to acquire information about making a change? See, that's a positive!

You don't need to have a last big blowout meal. You don't have to have a pity party. After all, if you'll remember, if you want to go by my theories put forth in this book, you don't really have to give up anything. You just have to learn to live within moderation and add some better choices.

Alternatives to your favorite foods exist. There are different ways to prepare the foods you've loved for years and so that they taste the same but are better for you. The same can be said for the way you see yourself. There's a different way to look at yourself and it's in a positive light.

And if there are others around you who do not shine that light of positive thinking on you, get rid of them. They are negative forces whether they realize it. If they don't or can't support your goals, consider them toxic. They bring stress and unhappiness and contribute to holding you back from your goals. I call them "toxic people."

If you are unhappy at your job and it's causing you to eat poorly or to feel a failure, think about what else you can do professionally. If you can't afford to leave the job, get involved in volunteer work in the community. Talk about gaining self worth...helping others enables you to see there are others who are less fortunate. What better way to boost you into sticking to your plans for success.

But, of course, you must be realistic about what you intend to accomplish. I know I'll never wear slacks with a 32-inch waist so I'm not working toward that. I mainly just want to be comfortable with my looks and my health.

It will take about six weeks for you to feel significantly better physically. But the first day of your new life should provide a boost of pride and positivity that you are taking control and turning yourself into a happy, healthy individual. Bask in that momentum and you'll see how you will continue to feel better and be better.

Chill Out

Do minor mishaps such as misplacing things, traffic jams, missed appointments, unreturned phone calls tick you off big time? Do you start throwing things? If so, I consider you a candidate for a primary coronary; the big one. It all relates to and is caused by stress. You know it and maybe you feel like there's not much you can do about it. One good heart attack will change your mind, real quick.

You can be the thinnest chap or gal in town, but if you're stressed out, you're in the same bad shape as someone who needs to lose weight. Long hours, bad tempers, and too much fat all tear at our bodies, outside and inside.

And if you think you're not affected by these common irritations and that you don't demonstrate an ugly side of your personality, try recalling the last time you were trapped in traffic at five in the afternoon. Honking, yelling, cussing and flapping your fingers at those around you who were trapped in their own vehicles wasn't pretty at all. That's not nice behavior and it's not good for you. You don't even really feel better after making all of those complicated gestures and forming those bad words, now do you?

It's time to chill out, cool off and calm down. You can teach yourself to do that, just as you can train yourself to eat healthier and feel better. I have come quite a long way from that fast track. When someone cuts me off, I let it go. It just doesn't matter. You can't get to your destination any sooner.

What can make you feel good is when you learn that when you display kindness, people around you aren't sure what to make of your actions. Once while driving, I accidentally cut another motorist off. As he viciously signaled his digits at me, I pulled off and let him pass me and tipped my hat as he proceeded. This poor guy had no idea what I was doing and was completely baffled. His fingers grew silent. As I followed him, I watched as he suspiciously and continuously gazed at me in his rear view mirror. All in all it was amusing, not aggravating.

Like changing your eating habits, it's not easy changing the stresses in your life. But it can and should be done. You want to be healthy, right? That's why you're reading this. Think about what really sets you off and position it somewhere in your grand scheme of life. Not much room for it, is there? There's too much going on in your body on a regular basis for you to be goofing it up with stress.

The human heart pumps 2,100 gallons of blood a day. This seems like a full-time job to me. Don't be messing with that pump. Anger and stress just make it work faster and harder. Like your car, the more wear and tear, the fewer years your pump has ahead.

Options abound for getting mellow. Start by having your blood pressure checked. Then stop and smell the roses. If a bee stings you, put yourself in the place of that insect. What would you do if you saw a giant nose coming at you?

Life can be humorous. Make it fun. Give your fingers a rest from flipping out. Read a book, listen to music, take a bath. This is it folks, we don't get a second chance. Life is not a dress rehearsal.

Let's *Not* Do Lunch?

When Franklin D. Roosevelt said we had nothing to fear but fear itself, he obviously had not perceived the power of a pastrami on rye. Something as innocent looking as a sandwich, the traditional food stuff of the noon hour, has made more than one cry out, "I don't want to do lunch, I'm afraid!"

"Doing lunch" or dinner means eating in public, in a restaurant, an activity that can ignite raw, hard-core terror in those who are diligently watching their weight. The thought of being taunted by a glass-encased display of pastries slowly spinning and teasing outsiders is enough to keep some from even entering a Howard Johnson's to use the restroom.

It was my very own mother who when invited to dine out at midday, declined and candidly admitted, "I'm not strong." She had been actively involved in a war with her weight and did not want to lose a single battle. She was scared to risk being tempted by the servers lugging lusciously loaded trays of desserts, waving them from side to side in front of their patrons' faces. She knew she could be knocked into caloric hell by the server's toss of a chocolate mint candy as Mom was preparing to tip.

Eating out can make you feel as if you've lost complete control and handed yourself over to a huge restaurant chain for management to do as it pleases. But I'm here to tell you that it doesn't have to be that way. You can do whatever the heck you want. You just have to learn how.

It's imporant that you learn to choose the right restaurant, specifically one with a real chef instead of an eatery operating with "clipboard cooks," the kind of food preparers who know how to open cans rather than how to invent a meal.

If management is concerned whether you enjoy your meal, it will try to accommodate your dining requests. I know, because I had my own restaurant and I'm a nice guy. I was always willing to help someone's dietary needs. I wanted them to want to come back to my establishment, and they did.

Selecting a restaurant that has your needs and pleasures at heart takes more than smarts on your part; it requires guts. You must have the courage to leave if the management isn't willing to try to meet your requests. You don't have to steamroll over the serving staff and screech out insults about the food as you leave. You must be able to excuse yourself politely and try another establishment where you get food prepared according to your requirements. After all, eating out is supposed to be about you getting what you want and being satisfied.

The best way to determine whether a restaurant will cooperate is to ask. Isn't that easy? You can interrogate the servers, the hostess, the manager; someone working there should be able to answer your questions. You might want to know if you can get a sauce served on the side, whether salt is used in a particular dish, will the chef leave it out at your request, does the restaurant poach food, is broiling available, can vegetables be steamed? You have the right to ask. You have the need to ask.

Don't be embarrassed and stay if the answers aren't what you want. Get up and leave. That's why you asked in the first place. In fact, more people should do this so restaurants sharpen their wits and culinary skills to please more patrons.

But there is more that you must do to make eating out fun and fearless. Veer away from the rich sauces, heavy entrees and desserts that tease you as you read the menu. I know how I am. I love the way certain foods smell, feel and taste and once they are made known to me, they're pretty hard to resist. However, I also know how I feel after I've overindulged and that's not so hot. Not only do I feel bad that I gave in when I shouldn't have, but since I've gotten healthier, my body doesn't react well to these riches so I'm physically bothered as well as emotionally. And, of course, then I think of "D-I-E-T" and I ask myself in amazement, "Did I Eat That?"

Getting through a meal away from your own kitchen can be accomplished with a great deal of fun. Like every good soldier in combat, (and yes, this is a war), you should equip yourself so that you are prepared to win this and every battle. Like the finest fighting troops, I carry special gear with me; I've been doing it for years and it works.

When I "do lunch," I pack lunch, sort of. I've been carrying everything from spices to cheeses into restaurants of all levels and have never had a problem. Even when Ellen and I go for pizza, we ask the pizza man to use cheese that we bring and to ease up on the oil and hold the salt. He is happy to prepare the pie our way. We eat there regularly and he accommodates us gladly.

There is no limit to what you can pack in your "survival kit." I've carried oregano, powdered garlic, cayenne pepper, balsamic vinegar, hot sauce, Sap Sago cheese and the kitchen sink (okay, not really, but you get the picture). You just can't be concerned with what others think as they watch you actively participate in the preparation of your meal. In fact, they'll probably be impressed that you had the chutzpah to take such control.

It doesn't matter what you use to schlep your supplies, just pack up in whatever makes you comfortable. A salad dressing company that has been advertising its fat-free product on television, shows a woman who carries a bottle or two of the stuff in a big handbag. Very trendy.

Other issues invade the event of eating out. You may have the best intentions when your co-workers team up and head to the joint across the street for lunch and gossip. You know that everything's fine when you refrain from ordering dessert. But when the guy sitting next to you asks for apple pie a la mode, and the office secretary chooses mud pie, your resistance is piqued. Peer pressure can ruin all the best intentions in the world. Be strong. Don't order dessert if you know you shouldn't have it.

Then there's the problem of attending parties and other functions revolving around food. Alcohol, for instance, can hamper dining out if you let it. Not only does it mess up your driving, it can mess up your healthy eating regimen if you cave in. Alcoholic beverages are steeped with calories.

People often order drinks they wouldn't make at home just because it's fun and the concoctions are tasty. But requesting a coconut or tropical punch with an umbrella and foliage hanging out are bad choices, very bad. They may be great to look at, but they'll hang on you lots longer than that sprig of grass did on your glass.

A better choice is to ask for a wine spritzer. If the establishment doesn't make them, once again, take charge. Request a glass of wine and a bottle of Perrier on the side. Mix them yourself. And make it last a long time so you don't order another. Let me take this opportunity to say that you don't need alcohol to be sociable. You can still enjoy a meal out by imbibing in a glass of mineral or Perrier water adorned with a twist of lemon.

Another dining dilemma is breakfast, which has become very popular at restaurants. Breakfast is more important than the others because it's what gets your body started each day and it shouldn't be skipped.

Although searching for a salad bar at lunch or dinner times is a good idea, eating from a breakfast bar isn't. Besides often being expensive, these displays offer unhealthy servings of cholesterol, sugar and fat, fat, fat. And because there is so much food on site, people tend to eat more with their eyes than their mouths by loading up on more food than they would or should normally consume. I have found that most restaurants with a breakfast menu or bar also offer cereal. The problem is milk. Most restaurants serve it whole and that's too much fat. If you can't get skim and don't want to bring it with you try this trick. Have your cereal with water. If you close your eyes you can't tell the difference. You also can't see where you're putting your spoon so here's an alternative to my alternative. Choose a cereal with low or no fat content. Since restaurants usually serve whole milk, mix a spoonful of milk with a spoonful of water and voila! If you're lucky you can get a banana or some other fresh fruit to top it off.

Hot cereals like oatmeal also are a tasty and safe option as are pancakes if adorned properly. For flapjacks, you must remember either to bring your own fresh fruit, all fruit jelly, or lite maple syrup rather than rely on the restaurant to provide a topping that's low-cal, sugar or fat free.

If you're uneasy about grilling the restaurant as to whether the staff will take any special measures for your meal, there's always the standard — the salad bar. Just about everyone can always find something there.

Salad bars range from the most basic to a virtual farm setting offering a bountiful display that includes a variety of fresh raw vegetables, baked potatoes, hot vegetables, soups and fresh bread. In the better establishments, a salad bar can include pure fruit sorbet. (This is different from sherbet, which contains cream or milk; sorbet is just the sugar and flavorings.) Another popular item often accompanying salad bars is non-fat yogurt, God's gift to the world. Oh yes, this has saved me many times.

It may be tough training your mind to want frozen yogurt instead of your favorite rum raisin ice cream, but there are ways around all dilemmas. I once made a "safe" rum raisin sauce to be used with frozen yogurt, so you see there are acceptable alternatives. You have to be open-minded and somewhat adventurous.

And speaking of open-minded, don't forget that the above mentioned tips, such as the survival kit, can be applied when you travel on business or vacation. It just takes some planning on your part, which you have to do anyway.

Now you know, you CAN do lunch, dinner, breakfast or whatever you want. You're already one step ahead of the rest of the world by reading this book and making these changes in your eating habits. While you actively pursue requiring restaurants to prepare your meals so they are healthy, many establishments are taking steps themselves by using less fat, steaming vegetables and cutting out salt. New recipes are being created every day to provide healthier options for diners.

You will find that restaurants willing to accommodate your special requests, will continue to do so when they see you return. Just don't be afraid. You can get what you want, the way you want it. I just say, "Please help me for I'm trying to get thin and handsome." So, yes, Let's Do Lunch!

Hints & Tips

You've been hinting about losing weight because you're tipping the scales so here are some real hints and tips that can help you get thin and handsome as well as healthy and happier about yourself. I'm sure some of these you've heard before and maybe even tried. I can tell you this, these "tricks" work, so don't take them lightly.

- Write It Down. Keep a notebook of everything you eat. The power of the pen may overcome the power of the snack. And if not, reading about what you ate yesterday will paint a vivid picture. You can be the Ernest Hemingway of weight loss by maintaining a journal. Write down absolutely everything. It's like keeping a personal scoreboard that lets you tally up points for eating more of the right stuff and less of the bad. If you attempt a little Creative Writing 101 by embellishing or leaving out facts, you'll know the truth so you won't be fooling your reader.

- Lighten Up the Refrigerator. Install a blue bulb. What was the last blue food you ate? And I don't mean that sad-looking container of leftovers. I'm talking the color blue. Other than berries, you probably haven't. There's a reason for that. Humans are put off by edible items that are the same color as the sky. Would you care for a glass of blue milk? I don't think so. Therefore, I make my point; a blue haze hanging over the contents of your refrigerator will curb your appetite.

- Never Go Hungry — Especially To the Grocery Store. That's the time when everything looks delicious and you begin to buy STUFF; the items you wouldn't normally buy or eat. It's just that if you're hungry that urge takes control of your common sense and your shopping cart. The key is to plan ahead, make a list of the items you need and stick to that. Not only will you save on fat and calories, but you'll save on your grocery bill, too. Junk food is expensive!

- Relax and Slow Your Fork From Warp Speed. You can always try to eat slower, or eat with a shrimp cocktail fork, but that takes a lot of effort. Here's an idea that has worked for me time and again. When you sit at the table, place both feet flat on the floor, place one hand on each knee, sit back in your chair, relax, close your eyes and take in seven very deep breaths and slowly exhale. This has a terrific calming effect and slows down your eating. You're so busy trying not to hyperventilate that the meal becomes less important.

- Flush It Out. This is an old standard that everyone's heard about. Drink at least eight, eight ounce glasses of water a day and try to have one before each meal to give you that full feeling. You'll consume smaller portions of food. This flood of water helps you flush fat out of your system. And think of all the exercise you'll get as you trot back and forth to the bathroom.

- Don't Give Up — I don't want you to give up on healthy eating, but I also don't want you to deny yourself the foods you enjoy. If you do, you're sure to break down at some point and binge and then you'll really feel terrible. Remember earlier in this book how I said to take one day off and just enjoy yourself. You don't have to go overboard, but just enjoy some of the things you like. Go ahead and have the piece of candy or that big old cowboy steak. Just don't do this daily or every other day. Be disciplined, and jump back on the system.

- Don't Dream The Impossible — I know what I'll never look like. I'm never going to look like Paul Newman. My eyes aren't the right color. All I want is to be healthy and to reach a comfortable weight that's not too much for my heart to manage and a body that can be adorned in an off-the-rack wardrobe. I've already reached that point and will continue to trim down a bit more.

- Don't set unreasonable goals. So what if you don't get stick thin like Cher. You'd have to get a couple tattoos anyway and that would hurt. So just realize that you want to be healthy and comfortable and you've set an attainable goal; one that when reached will make you feel like you've really accomplished something special, which will be true.

- Replace Your Place — This is simple enough. First start by ditching all the "bad" foods — give them to the neighbor or the homeless shelter. Just get the poison out of the cupboards and fridge. Now you're ready to shop correctly and healthfully. Make the switch. Replace butter with margarine, and replace margarine with apple butter or pure fruit jellies. Switch ground beef recipes with ground turkey. Switch the whole milk with skim. Change the mayonnaise with non-fat mayonnaise. When reading recipes learn to switch high fat ingredients with healthier substitutes. Don't switch salt, just stop using it.

    I'm telling you, I've been doing all of this for a couple of years now and it does work.

- Start Cookin' In The Kitchen. When I say "cookin'," I mean "COOKIN'." Start thinking like a chef and become the master of your kitchen. Make all this food preparation fun. Get yourself the right tools. Get an inexpensive food processor, a couple of good knives, some funky looking wall hangings and make the kitchen the place to hang out, to cook, to entertain. That's usually where everybody ends up anyway.

    Operate under the same theory as you do in your office or your place of work. You probably have an electric pencil sharpener, an answering machine, or a computer. These are all designed to make your work more efficient and easier to perform. So do the same in the kitchen. Browse the flea markets, yard sales and antique shops for funky dishware and interesting decorations for your table settings. And when you fix a meal, dress it up with some paper umbrellas, some parsley, anything that makes your meal more attractive and more entertaining. The difference between work and your kitchen is that cooking is meant to be fun.

In Conclusion...

If you have taken the time to read my book, you are on your way to being well. Remember, the longest journey begins with a single first step. It's not easy, but if you've really made up your mind, that step is the start of a new and better way of life.

Don't wait until Monday, which may be a day or two after tomorrow, because yesterday is already here today. Do these things for yourself and you'll find that those around you will benefit, too. You may be surprised when you meet the new you that emerges. It's a rocky road at first with temptations to dodge. Be persistent and never, never give up. You are a winner.

I wish you the best.

"Lite-en" up,

RECIPES

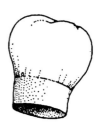

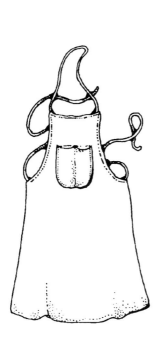

APPETIZERS

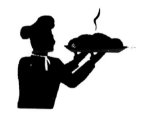

FRESH RAW VEGGIES
YOGURT CHEESE
HOOP CHEESE
EGGPLANT DIP
TROPICAL FRUIT CHUTNEY
CAESAR DIP
SALSA - PICANTE
HUMMUS DIP
CURRY DIP
ONION DIP

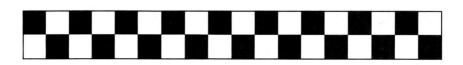

Raw Veggies

Nothing like fresh raw vegetables — low in calories, high in fiber and essential vitamins and minerals. Keep plenty cut at all times. Serve plain or with a dip. Here are a few veggie suggestions for a nice platter.

Asparagus Spears
Green Onions
Broccoli Florets
Mushrooms
Carrot Sticks
Pepper Strips — Red, Green & Yellow
Cauliflower Florets
Radishes
Celery Sticks
Snow Peas
Cucumber Slices
Tomatoes — Cherry or Slices
Green Onions
Yellow Squash
Zucchini Slices

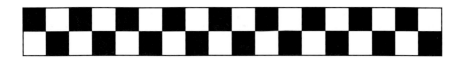

Yogurt Cheese

2 Cups Non-Fat Yogurt

     Line a strainer with about 3 layers of cheesecloth. Pour in yogurt and place strainer over container to drain overnight in refrigerator. The curd that remains in the cheesecloth is just like cream cheese.
YIELDS 1 CUP
NOTE: Yogurt strainers are available in kitchen and health food stores.

NUTRITIONAL ANALYSIS
Per 1 Tbsp. Portion

Calories	10	Protein	1 gm
Fat	0 gm	Carbohydrate	1 gm
Sodium	10 mg	Cholesterol	0 mg

Hoop Cheese

1 Cup Low-Fat Cottage Cheese
  Fine Mesh Strainer

     Place low-fat cottage cheese in fine mesh strainer and rinse all the whey off the curds under cold running water. Drain thoroughly. Hoop cheese is what remains.
YIELDS 1 CUP

NUTRITIONAL ANALYSIS
Per Cup Portion
Hoop cheese cannot as yet be accurately analyzed, but the amounts are significantly less than stated on the cottage cheese container.

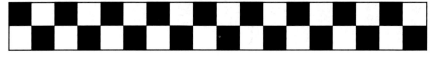

Eggplant Dip

1 Large Eggplant (about 1½ pounds)
¼ Cup Port Wine
2 Tablespoons Olive Oil
½ Cup Skim Milk
2 teaspoons White Vinegar
¼ Cup Low-Fat Cottage Cheese
1 Clove Garlic-Minced (optional)
4 Drops Tabasco Sauce or To Taste

In an 8-quart dutch oven, submerge whole unpeeled eggplant into boiling water and boil for 20 minutes. Carefully remove from water and let cool. (It will shrivel.) Cut off stem and discard. Cut remaining eggplant into pieces small enough to fit into processor. Process until creamy. Add the rest of the ingredients and process until satin smooth. Serve as a dip for vegetables cut into strips such as carrots, peppers, celery, zucchini, etc. YIELDS 2 CUPS

NUTRITIONAL ANALYSIS
Per 1 Tbsp. Portion

Calories	18	Protein	less than 1 gm
Fat	less than 1 gm	Carbohydrate	2 gm
Sodium	10 mg	Cholesterol	less than 1 mg

Tropical Fruit Chutney

1 15¼ oz. Can Tropical Fruit Cocktail — Reserve Liquid!
2 Tablespoons Orange Juice Concentrate
¼ Cup Apple Cider Vinegar
1 Tablespoon Cornstarch
1 Small Onion — Chopped
2 Tablespoons Fresh Ground Ginger
¼ Cup Raisins
1 or 2 Cloves Garlic — Minced
1 Tablespoon Lemon Zest (Fresh is Best)
1 Tablespoon Molasses
  Cayenne Pepper to Taste, ¼ to ½ tsp. if you like it hot!

Open can of Tropical Fruits, but save liquid. Set fruits aside. Put orange juice concentrate, vinegar and cornstarch in a small bowl and mix until smooth. Set aside. Pour reserved Tropical Fruit liquid into saucepan and add onion, ginger, raisins, garlic, lemon zest, molasses and cayenne pepper. Bring to boil and cook 2 to 3 minutes stirring constantly. Now add orange juice concentrate mixture to boiling mixture and stir until smooth, about 30 seconds. Add Tropical Fruits, mixing well. Chill and Serve.

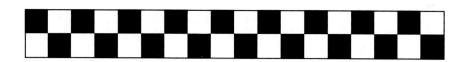

YIELDS ABOUT 2 CUPS
NOTE: This chutney is a great accompaniment to most dishes such as lamb, curry, fish, chicken, etc. Try it with crackers as an appetizer.

NUTRITIONAL ANALYSIS
Per 2 Tbsp. Portion

Calories	42	Protein	less than 1 gm
Fat	Less than 1 gm	Carbohydrate	11 gm
Sodium	5 mg	Cholesterol	0 mg

Caesar Dip

1¼ Cup Cottage Cheese (Low-Fat)
¼ Cup No Cholesterol Low-Fat Mayonnaise
3 teaspoons Anchovy Paste
2 Cloves Garlic
1 teaspoon Dry Mustard Powder
2 teaspoons White Vinegar
¼ teaspoon Black Pepper
    Pinch of Cayenne Pepper

    Place all above ingredients in a processor and blend until velvety smooth.
MAKES 1¼ CUPS

NUTRITIONAL ANALYSIS
Per 1 Tbsp. Portion

Calories	23	Protein	2 gm
Fat	1 gm	Carbohydrate	less than 1 gm
Sodium	106 mg	Cholesterol	1 mg

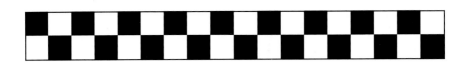

Salsa-Picante

2 Tomatoes — chopped
1 Onion — chopped
1 Green Bell Pepper — chopped
2 Stalks Celery — chopped
1 4 oz. Can Chopped Green Chiles
½ Cup White Vinegar
1 Tablespoon Cilantro or Parsley
1 teaspoon Oregano
1 Tablespoon Chili Powder
Cayenne or Red Pepper to Taste

1 or 2 Jalapeños to Taste with seeds removed; if using canned jalapeños, rinse well and remove seeds.
5½ oz. Can of V8 or Tomato Juice (low salt)
3 Tablespoons Cornstarch
1 Tablespoon Sugar
5 Cloves Garlic — minced
1 Tablespoon Paprika

Place all ingredients in a saucepan and bring to a boil stirring constantly. Reduce heat, simmer 4 minutes stirring constantly. Remove from heat, chill and enjoy. Hot, spicy and unforgettable!!!

NUTRITIONAL ANALYSIS
Per 1 oz. Portion

Calories	13	Protein	less than 1 gm
Fat less than	1 gm	Carbohydrate	3 gm
Sodium	29 mg	Cholesterol	less than 1 mg

Hummus Dip

1 15 oz. Can Garbanzo Beans — rinsed and drained
2 Tablespoons Lemon Juice
2 Tablespoons Red Wine Vinegar
2 Tablespoons Port Wine or Apple Juice
1-2 Cloves Garlic Minced (more if you like garlic)
¼ Cup Dry Parsley
1 teaspoon Oregano
⅛ teaspoon Cayenne Pepper

Put all ingredients in food processor and blend until mixture is smooth. Be patient. If mixture is too thick, add 1 to 2 tablespoons of water to obtain desired consistency.
YIELDS 1 CUP

NUTRITIONAL ANALYSIS
Per 1 Tbsp. Portion

Calories	36	Protein	1 gm
Fat	less than 1 gm	Carbohydrate	7 gm
Sodium	80 mg	Cholesterol	0 mg

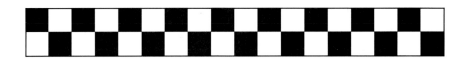

Curry Dip

1 Cup Hoop Cheese (Refer to Hoop Cheese Recipe in this section)
1 8 oz. Can Pineapple Chunks — thoroughly drained
1 teaspoon Curry Powder
2 teaspoons Prepared Mustard (Dijon)
¼ teaspoon Cayenne Pepper (½ tsp. if you like it hot)

Place all above ingredients in food processor and process until smooth. Chill and serve.
YIELDS 1½ CUPS

NUTRITIONAL ANALYSIS
Per 1 Tbsp. Portion

Calories	14	Protein	1 gm
Fat	less than 1 gm	Carbohydrate	2 gm
Sodium	51 mg	Cholesterol	less than 1 mg

Onion Dip

1 Cup Hoop Cheese* (Refer to Hoop Cheese Recipe in this section)
1 Medium Onion — sliced
1 teaspoon Vegetable oil
3 Green Onions — cut into 1 inch pieces including green tops
1 Tablespoon Dry Parsley
1 teaspoon Oregano
1 teaspoon White Vinegar
  Drop of Hot Sauce to Taste

Saute onions in vegetable oil, in a 10" non-stick skillet until golden brown. Place in processor with hoop cheese and the rest of the ingredients. Process until smooth. Chill 1 to 2 hours.
YIELDS 1½ CUPS

NUTRITIONAL ANALYSIS
Per 1 Tbsp. Portion

Calories	10	Protein	1 gm
Fat	less than 1 gm	Carbohydrate	1 gm
Sodium	less than 1 mg	Cholesterol	less than 1 mg

BREAKFAST IDEAS

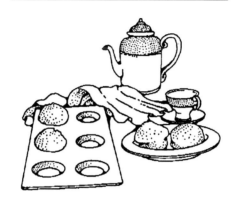

BRAN AND OATS BAKING MIX
BRAN AND OATS CINNAMON PANCAKES
BRAN AND OATS CARROT MUFFINS
BRAN AND OATS SPICED ZUCCHINI
COFFEE CAKE
BRAN AND OATS APPLE MUFFINS

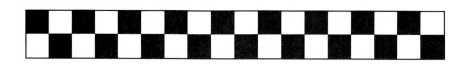

Breakfast

You've heard it before so I'll say it again. This is the most important meal of the day. It's because your blood sugar is very low and your body (and probably your mind) is in low gear.

This isn't a green light to chow down on bacon, eggs, hash browns and all that stuff. (You've read too far into this book to think that.)

You have to change those eating habits and you might as well start with breakfast. And don't think you have to wait until Monday to get cranking. There's no logic in waiting until then, and it's a big reason why weight loss programs fail; people wait too long.

If you start with a good (and by good I mean nutritious) breakfast, you won't feel pooped by 10 a.m. and head for the nearest doughnut shop for a snack.

The smartest thing you could do to begin your healthy breakfast pattern is to reduce how much COFFEE you drink each morning. Meanwhile, fresh fruit juice, perhaps mixed with sparkling water is a refreshing way to start. Breakfast gets even better when you add hot or cold cereals. (Be sure to read the label and make sure you've omitted the salt.) If cereal's not for you, try whole grain toast with yogurt cheese in place of cream cheese and you might even add a little pure fruit jelly. Another choice that's delicious and healthy is a ripe banana spread on a bagel with a little jelly.

If you'd rather purchase a commercially prepared muffin, just be sure to read the label and make sure the ingredients are acceptable.

Then watch how perky you'll be all morning. You'll be amazed and you'll be awake.

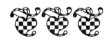

Bran and Oats Baking Mix

1½ Cups Flour
½ Cup Whole Wheat Flour
1 Cup Miller's Bran
1 Cup Quick Oats
½ Cup Sugar
2 Tablespoons Featherlite Baking Powder or 1 Tablespoon of Regular Baking Powder

Place all above ingredients in a large bowl and mix until well-blended. Store in an air-tight container until needed.
YIELDS 4 CUPS

NUTRITIONAL ANALYSIS
Per 1 Cup Portion

Calories	440	Protein	12 gm
Fat	3 gm	Carbohydrate	98 gm
Sodium	3 mg	Cholesterol	0 mg

Bran and Oats Cinnamon Pancakes

Cups Bran & Oats Baking Mix (See Recipe)
3 Egg Whites
1 Cup Water
1 teaspoon Cinnamon
½ teaspoon Vegetable Oil per Cooking Batch

Put all ingredients in a medium bowl and beat with a whisk or electric beater until smooth. Lightly oil a 12″, non-stick skillet and preheat over medium-high heat. Pour a little less than ¼ cup of batter for each pancake. Pour measured batter in skillet (2 pancakes will fit in 12″ pan) and cook for 1½-2 minutes or until mixture starts to bubble. Turn each cake over and cook 1½-2 minutes longer. Pour one of my dessert syrups, low calorie syrup or sprinkle powdered sugar on top and enjoy.
MAKES 9 PANCAKES; SERVES 4

NUTRITIONAL ANALYSIS
Per 1 Each Portion (1 Pancake)

Calories	111	Protein	4 gm
Fat	1 gm	Carbohydrate	22 gm
Sodium	19 mg	Cholesterol	0 mg

Bran and Oats Carrot Muffins

1 Cup Bran & Oats Baking Mix (See Recipe)
3 Tablespoons 1% Buttermilk or Skim Milk
2 Egg Whites
2 teaspoons Vegetable Oil
1 Tablespoon Brown Sugar
¾ Cup Carrots — peeled and very finely shredded
  Non-stick Cooking Spray

    Preheat oven to 375 degrees.
    Place all ingredients in a medium bowl and beat with a whisk until smooth. Spoon into muffin pan lined with paper muffin cups that have been lightly sprayed with non-stick cooking spray. Bake at 375 degrees for 20 minutes.
MAKES 6 MUFFINS

NUTRITIONAL ANALYSIS
Per Portion

Calories	112	Protein	4 gm
Fat	2 gm	Carbohydrate	21 gm
Sodium	33 mg	Cholesterol	less than 1 mg

Bran and Oats Spiced Zucchini Coffee Cake

2 Cups Bran and Oats Baking Mix (See Recipe)
1 Cup Zucchini — shredded
½ Cup 1% Buttermilk or Skim Milk
3 Egg Whites
1 teaspoon Pumpkin Pie Spice
  Non-Stick Cooking Spray
¼ teaspoon Allspice, Optional
1 Tablespoon Powdered Sugar, Optional

    Preheat oven to 375 degrees.
    Put Bran and Oats Baking Mix, shredded zucchini, buttermilk, egg whites and pumpkin pie spice in a medium bowl and beat with a whisk until smooth. Spray a 9" cake pan lightly with non-stick cooking spray and pour in the batter. Bake in a 375 degree oven for 20 to 25 minutes.
OPTIONAL: Mix allspice and powdered sugar together and dust on top of cake after removing from pan before serving.
SERVES 8

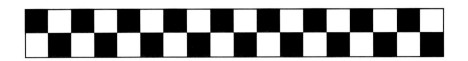

NUTRITIONAL ANALYSIS
Per Portion

Calories	112	Protein	4 gm
Fat	2 gm	Carbohydrate	21 gm
Sodium	33 mg	Cholesterol	less than 1 mg

Bran and Oats Apple Muffins

1 Cup Bran & Oats Baking Mix (See Recipe)
3 Tablespoons Apple Juice
2 Egg Whites
2 teaspoons Vegetable Oil
1 Tablespoon Molasses
1 teaspoon Apple Pie Spice
¾ Cup Apples — Peeled, Cored and Chopped
   Non-Stick Cooking Spray

Preheat oven to 375 degrees.
Place all ingredients in a medium bowl and beat with a whisk until smooth. Spoon into a muffin pan bowl lined with paper muffin cups that have been lightly sprayed with non-stick cooking spray. Fill ¾ full.
YIELDS 6 MUFFINS

NUTRITIONAL ANALYSIS
Per Portion

Calories	114	Protein	3 gm
Fat	2 gm	Carbohydrate	22 gm
Sodium	20 mg	Cholesterol	0 mg

VEGGIE SANDWICH

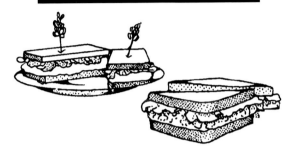

Veggie Sandwich

½ Cup Tomatoes — diced
½ Cup Onions — chopped
½ Cup Zucchini — shredded
½ Cup Carrots — finely shredded
½ Cup Green Bell Pepper — chopped
½ Cup Broccoli — chopped
¼ Cup Honey Mustard Dressing (see Dressings section)

Place all ingredients in a medium mixing bowl and mix until well blended. Stuff in pita pockets with shredded lettuce.
SERVES 4

This Veggie Sandwich is just a basic combination. If you don't like onions, don't use them — no one will care. Chop up some cucumbers instead. Get the idea? These recipes are not prescriptions. To this basic Veggie Sandwich a lot can be done. Add tuna, beef, pork, beans or whatever. Be creative and maybe you'll send me a recipe.

SOUPS & CHOWDERS

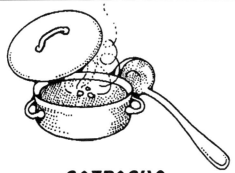

GAZPACHO
CORN AND PEPPER CHOWDER
ARTHUR'S VEGERAMA
TOMATO RICE SOUP
GREEN CHILE SOUP
LIGHT CLAM CHOWDER
VEGETABLE SOUP
CURRIED POTATO LEEK SOUP

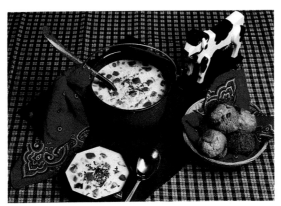

Corn & Pepper
Chowder

Bran & Oats
Apple Muffins

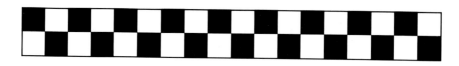

Soups

I like soups because they take a long time to eat and when you eat slowly it gives your blood sugar a chance to rise and you start to feel full sooner. (Remember that kid in the school cafeteria who took forever to finish lunch? Odds are that kid never had a weight problem.)

Not only do soups take a while to eat, they are economical and nutritious.

The safest way to appreciate soup is to avoid commercially prepared soups, which contain too much salt. While there are some good ones on the market, take some time to experiment with these recipes and taste the difference.

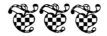

Gazpacho

3 Tomatoes — peeled and chopped
1 Cucumber — peeled, seeded and chopped
½ Green Bell Pepper — seeded and chopped
1 Small Onion — chopped
4 Green Onions — chopped
2-3 Cloves Garlic — minced
3 Stalks Celery — chopped
2 Tablespoons Parsley (dry will do)
3 Tablespoons Lemon Juice
3 Tablespoons White Vinegar
2 Cups V8 or Tomato Juice (no salt added)
2 teaspoons Paprika
¼ teaspoon Chili Powder
¼ teaspoon Celery Seed
¼ teaspoon Oregano
¼ teaspoon Thyme
  Touch of Cayenne Pepper

Place all ingredients in a blender. Pulsate blender until all ingredients have reached desired consistency. May be served pureed or chunky according to taste. Chill for 2 hours before serving.
SERVES 6-8

NUTRITIONAL ANALYSIS
Per Portion

Calories	43	Protein	2 gm
Fat	Less than 1 gm	Carbohydrate	10 gm
Sodium	254 mg	Cholesterol	0 mg

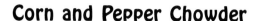

Corn and Pepper Chowder

2 Cups Whole Kernel Corn (fresh, frozen or canned)
2 Bell Peppers — 1 red, 1 green — seeded and coarsely chopped
1 Medium Onion — coarsely chopped
2 Cloves Garlic — minced
1 teaspoon Low-Sodium Chicken Broth Granules
   Pinch of Black Pepper
½ teaspoon Liquid Smoke (optional, but tasty)
2½ Cups Water
1 Tablespoon Chopped Parsley (dry will do)
1 teaspoon Oregano
1½ Cups Water
¼ Cup Low-Fat Ricotta Cheese
2 Tablespoons Cornstarch

Place all but the last 3 ingredients (1½ cups water, ricotta cheese and cornstarch) in a large soup pot. Bring to a boil stirring constantly. Cook for 8 to 10 minutes. Meanwhile put the 1½ cups water, ¼ cup ricotta cheese and 2 Tbs. cornstarch in a blender. Blend until very smooth — about 1 minute. After soup pot mixture has boiled for 10 minutes, add the blended ricotta cheese mixture to the soup pot stirring constantly. Bring this mixture to a boil, reduce heat and simmer for 2 minutes. Soup is ready. YIELDS 4-5 CUPS

NUTRITIONAL ANALYSIS
Per Portion

Calories	127	Protein	5 gm
Fat	2 gm	Carbohydrate	24 gm
Sodium	35 mg	Cholesterol	5 mg

Arthur's Vegerama
(A SOUPerior Meal)

6 Cups Vegetable Stock
2 Medium Yellow Squash (¾ pound) — finely shredded
3 Carrots — peeled and finely shredded
1 Red Bell Pepper — chopped
1 Green Bell Pepper — chopped
8 Green Onions — chopped
1 15-Oz. Container Low-Fat Ricotta Cheese
¾ Cup Water
⅓ Cup Flour
1 16-Oz. Bag Frozen Mixed Vegetables (carrots, peas, corn, green beans, lima beans)

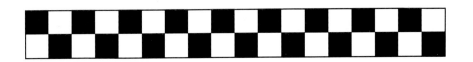

Place vegetable stock in a large soup pot with yellow squash, carrots, red bell peppers, green bell peppers and green onions. Over high heat bring to a boil. Place the ricotta cheese, water and flour in a blender and blend until smooth. Pour this mixture into vegetable stock. Blend in evenly with a whisk. Add frozen mixed vegetables and bring soup to a boil stirring occasionally. Over medium heat cook for about 15 minutes. Serve with fresh ground pepper.
SERVES 6-8

NUTRITIONAL ANALYSIS
Per Portion

Calories	158	Protein	13 gm
Fat	3 gm	Carbohydrate	23 gm
Sodium	803 mg	Cholesterol	6 mg

Tomato Rice Soup

1 28 oz. Can Crushed Tomatoes
3 Ripe Tomatoes — chopped
1 Medium Onion — chopped
½ Cup Dry Rice
2 Cloves Garlic — minced
½ teaspoon Basil
¼ teaspoon Thyme
½ teaspoon Chili Powder
  Pinch of Rosemary
  Touch of Black Pepper
6-7 Cups Water — start with 6 — more may be added*

Place all ingredients in a large soup pot. Bring to a boil over high heat stirring occasionally. Reduce heat, cover and simmer for 30 minutes or until rice is tender. Stir often so rice does not stick.
SERVES 6 to 8

* As the rice absorbs the liquid, more water may be added near the end of cooking.

NUTRITIONAL ANALYSIS
Per 1 Cup Portion

Calories	68	Protein	2 gm
Fat	less than 1 gm	Carbohydrate	15 gm
Sodium	9 mg	Cholesterol	0 mg

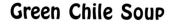

Green Chile Soup

2 Medium Onions — chopped
6 Green Onions — chopped (green tops also)
2 4 oz. Cans Green Chile Peppers — chopped
1-2 Cloves Garlic — minced
1 teaspoon Vegetable Broth Seasoning*
2½ Cups Water
½ teaspoon Chili Powder
¼ teaspoon Ground Cumin Seed
  Pinch of Cayenne Pepper (I use ⅛ tsp.) (optional)
  Pinch of Black Pepper (optional)
  Pinch of White Pepper (optional)
1½ Cups Water
¼ Cup Low-Fat Ricotta Cheese
1½ Tablespoon Cornstarch

Place all but the last 3 ingredients (1½ cups water, ricotta cheese and cornstarch) in a large soup pot. Bring to a boil, stirring constantly. Cook for 8 to 10 minutes. Meanwhile, put 1½ cups water, ¼ cup ricotta cheese and 1½ Tbs. cornstarch in a blender. Blend until very smooth, about 1 minute. After soup pot mixture has boiled for 10 minutes, add ricotta cheese mixture, stirring constantly. Bring this whole mixture to a boil, reduce heat and simmer for 2 minutes. Soup is ready.
YIELDS 4 CUPS
* Vegetable broth seasoning comes in granule or paste form and is available at most markets and health food stores.

NUTRITIONAL ANALYSIS
Per 1 Cup Portion

Calories	71	Protein	3 gm
Fat	1 gm	Carbohydrate	12 gm
Sodium	601 mg	Cholesterol	5 mg

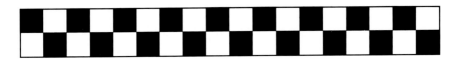

Light Clam Chowder

2½ Cups Chopped Clams (canned will do)
3 Cups Bottled Clam Juice
1 Cup Beer or Water
1 Medium Onion — chopped
1 Bay Leaf
1 Clove Garlic — minced
¼ teaspoon Thyme
¼ teaspoon Oregano
1½ Cups Diced Celery
¼ Cup Shredded Carrots
1½ Cups Diced Potatoes (½ inch dice)
4 Drops Tabasco Hot Sauce or to taste (optional)
   Black Pepper to Taste
2 Tablespoons Fresh Chopped Parsley

Combine clams, clam juice, beer or water, onion, bay leaf, garlic, thyme and oregano in a large soup pot. Over high heat bring to a boil. Reduce heat to medium, cover pot and simmer for 30 minutes. Add celery and carrots and cook 20 minutes longer. Add diced potatoes and cook another 20 minutes. Add optional hot sauce and pepper. Stir in chopped parsley and serve.
SERVES 6 to 8

NUTRITIONAL ANALYSIS
Per Portion

Calories	104	Protein	12 gm
Fat	less than 1 gm	Carbohydrate	12 gm
Sodium	295 mg	Cholesterol	28 mg

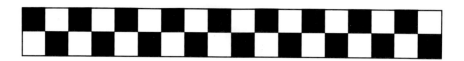

Vegetable Soup

3 Tomatoes — chopped
5 Cups Water
2 Carrots — diced
2 Celery Stalks — chopped (about ½ cup)
2 Medium Onions — chopped
¼ Head Cabbage — finely chopped
1 Medium Zucchini — chopped
1 Bell Pepper — seeded and chopped
2 Cloves Garlic — minced
1 Tablespoon Parsley
1 teaspoon Chili Powder
1 teaspoon Italian Seasoning
　 Touch of Pepper

　　　Put chopped tomatoes in a large soup pot with 5 cups of water. Bring to boil, reduce heat to medium and cook for 20 minutes. Add the rest of the ingredients, cover, reduce heat and simmer for 30 to 45 minutes more. SERVES 6

NUTRITIONAL ANALYIS
Per Portion

Calories	55	Protein	2 gm
Fat	less than 1 gm	Carbohydrate	12 gm
Sodium	36 mg	Cholesterol	0 mg

Curried Potato Leek Soup

5-8 Leeks (about 1 lb.) — cut off dark green tops and root ends
2-3 Medium Potatoes (about 1 lb.) — peeled and shredded
1 Medium Onion — chopped
1 Clove Garlic — chopped
¼ Cup Lemon Juice
3 Cups Chicken Stock (low-fat or low-sodium bouillon)
2 Cups Skim Milk
2 Cups Water
1 Tablespoon Curry Powder
¼ teaspoon Savory
¼ teaspoon Thyme

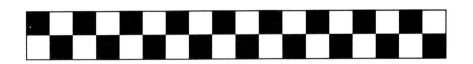

Wash and clean leeks thoroughly by splitting in half lengthwise. Rinse away all traces of sand and dirt near root end. Once cleaned, chop leeks into ½ inch pieces. Place all above ingredients in a large soup pot and bring to a boil. Cover and reduce heat to simmer. Cook for 30 to 35 minutes. Pour ½ or less of the cooked soup into a blender and blend until smooth.* Repeat blending process with remaining soup until all soup is blended. Return to pot, heat and serve.
YIELDS 4 CUPS

*Note: Be careful when blending hot liquids in a blender. Always start on low speed and never fill blender more than half. Hold top down with a towel.

NUTRITIONAL ANALYSIS
Per 1 Cup Portion

Calories	189	Protein	9 gm
Fat	2 gm	Carbohydrate	35 gm
Sodium	125 mg	Cholesterol	2 mg

SALADS

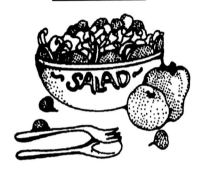

CALICO SALAD
GOLD COIN SALAD
CUCUMBER SALAD WITH YOGURT
CABBAGE SALAD
BEET AND ONION SALAD
WALDORF APPLE SALAD
MIDDLE EAST POTATO SALAD

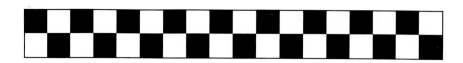

Calico Salad

2 Medium Carrots — peeled and diced (about 1 cup)
2 Cups Finely Chopped Fresh Spinach (about 6 ozs.)
1 16 oz. Can Whole Kernel Corn — rinsed and drained
1 Cucumber (about ¾ pound) — peeled, seeded and diced
2 Green Onions — chopped
1 Small Red Onion — chopped (about ¼ cup)
1 Prepared Recipe Creole Mustard Dressing (see Dressings)
½ Head Shredded Iceberg Lettuce (optional)

Prepare Creole Mustard Dressing. Set aside. Bring about 4 cups of water to a boil. When water is boiling pour in diced carrots. Cook about 2 minutes or until crisp tender. Remove from heat immediately, strain and rinse under cold water to stop the cooking. If you prefer a salad with more crunch, do not cook carrots. Combine all of the above ingredients along with cooked carrots and dressing in a large bowl. Toss gently until well blended. May be served over finely shredded lettuce if desired.
SERVES 6

NUTRITIONAL ANALYSIS
Per Portion

Calories	84	Protein	5 gm
Fat	1 gm	Carbohydrate	16 gm
Sodium	283 mg	Cholesterol	less than 1 mg

Gold Coin Salad

2 Pounds Large Carrots — peeled and cut into ¼ inch coins
1 Green Bell Pepper — seeded and cut into 2 inch long strips,
   ¼ inch wide
1 Medium Onion — sliced into paper-thin rings
2 Stalks Celery — diced
1 Prepared Recipe of Spicy Tomato Dressing (see Dressings)
½ Head Finely Shredded Lettuce if desired

Prepare Spicy Tomato Dressing and set aside. Place prepared carrots into a large pot of boiling water. Bring water to second rolling boil and cook carrots for 2 to 3 minutes or until crisp tender. Remove from heat, strain and rinse under cold water until cool. Put cooled carrots in a large bowl. Set aside. Add prepared dressing to the vegetables and toss lightly

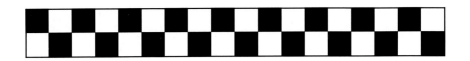

to blend well. Chill for 2 to 3 hours before serving. Serve about 1 cup of Gold Coin Salad per person over finely shredded lettuce if desired.
SERVES 6

NUTRITIONAL ANALYSIS
Per 1 Cup Portion

Calories	112	Protein	3 gm
Fat	less than 1 gm	Carbohydrate	26 gm
Sodium	225 mg	Cholesterol	0 mg

Cucumber Salad with Yogurt

2 Cucumbers — peeled and thinly sliced (⅛ - ¼ inch)
1 Red Onion — peeled and thinly sliced
1 Cup Non-Fat Yogurt
1 teaspoon Lemon Juice
1 teaspoon White Vinegar
1 Tablespoon Chopped Fresh Parsley (dry will do)
1 Tablespoon Chopped Fresh Mint (dry will do)

Place cucumbers and onion slices in a medium bowl. Mix remaining ingredients together in a separate bowl and pour over cucumbers and onions. Toss lightly and chill for 30 to 60 minutes. Gently toss again just before serving. Great in a pita pocket as a sandwich, too!
SERVES 4

NUTRITIONAL ANALYSIS
Per Portion

Calories	54	Protein	4 gm
Fat	less than 1 gm	Carbohydrate	9 gm
Sodium	46 mg	Cholesterol	1 mg

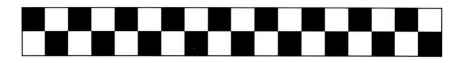

Cabbage Salad

4 Cups Finely Shredded Cabbage (about ½ a head)
¼ Cup Crumbled Feta Cheese — rinse thoroughly under water!
½ Cup Low-Fat Cottage Cheese
1 Tablespoon Grated Sap Sago Cheese or Grated Parmesan

DRESSING:
2 Tablespoons White Vinegar
  Juice of 1 Lemon
1 teaspoon Dill
1 teaspoon Parsley
½ teaspoon Oregano
½ Cup Non-Fat Yogurt

Mix all dressing ingredients together in a large bowl. Combine cabbage, rinsed Feta cheese, cottage cheese and Sap Sago or parmesan in a separate bowl and gently toss together. Transfer cabbage and cheese mixture into bowl of dressing and lightly toss together to thoroughly mix. Chill and toss lightly again just before serving. This salad is also great in a whole wheat pita pocket as a sandwich!
SERVES 4

NUTRITIONAL ANALYSIS
Per Portion

Calories	86	Protein	8 gm
Fat	2.5 gm	Carbohydrate	8 gm
Sodium	273 mg	Cholesterol	10 mg

Beet and Onion Salad

½ Pound Beets (young beets if possible). If using canned beets, rinse thoroughly under water
2 Medium Onions — coarsely chopped
½ Cup White Vinegar
¼ Cup Water
1 teaspoon Dill
1 teaspoon Oregano
1 teaspoon Prepared Horseradish
2 teaspoons Sugar

If using fresh beets, boil until tender (about 30 to 40 minutes). Peel and slice ⅛ to ¼ inch thick and allow to cool. If you are using canned beets, they are ready to go after being well-rinsed. If you are using whole canned beets, slice them ⅛ to ¼ inch thick. In a large bowl combine vinegar, water, dill, oregano, horseradish and sugar. Add beets and onions and toss lightly. Chill and serve.
SERVES 4

NUTRITIONAL ANALYSIS
Per Portion

Calories	45	Protein	1 gm
Fat	less than 1 gm	Carbohydrate	11 gm
Sodium	32 mg	Cholesterol	0 mg

Waldorf Apple Salad

*2 Apples Cored and Cut Into Small Pieces — about ½ inch cubes —
   I like to use 1 red and 1 green apple
1 Cup Diced Celery — about ½ inch pieces
1 Cup Seedless Red Grapes Cut in Half
1 8 oz. Can Water Chestnuts — drained and chopped into ¼ inch pieces
½ Cup Non-Fat Yogurt
2 Tablespoons No Cholesterol Mayonnaise
1 teaspoon Lemon Juice
   Touch of White Pepper

Combine all ingredients in a large bowl and toss lightly to mix well. Chill and serve.
SERVES 4

*When cutting apples, place the apple pieces in a bowl containing 1½ cups water and juice of 2 lemons. This will stop the apples from turning brown.

NUTRITIONAL ANALYSIS
Per Portion

Calories	83	Protein	2 gm
Fat	2 gm	Carbohydrate	17 gm
Sodium	62 mg	Cholesterol	less than 1 mg

Middle East Potato Salad

2 Pounds Potatoes — peeled, washed and cut into 1 inch cubes
1 Medium Onion — peeled, cut in half, thinly sliced
2 Cloves Garlic — minced
½ Cup Fresh Parsley — coarsely chopped
1 Tablespoon Dry Mint
1 teaspoon Oregano
   Pinch Cayenne Pepper
1 teaspoon Thyme
⅓ Cup Lemon Juice
2 Tablespoons Olive Oil
2 Tablespoons White Vinegar

Boil potatoes until firm but tender. Do not overcook! (Takes about 15 to 20 minutes). Cool by placing pot of potatoes in sink and running cold water gently over potatoes. Drain well when cool. Place remaining ingredients in a large bowl and mix well. Add cooked potatoes and toss gently to mix well. Serve.
SERVES 4 to 6

NUTRITIONAL ANALYSIS
Per Portion

Calories	157	Protein	3 gm
Fat	6 gm	Carbohydrate	25 gm
Sodium	14 mg	Cholesterol	0 mg

SALAD DRESSINGS

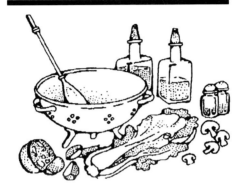

THOUSAND ISLAND DRESSING
SWEET AND SOUR TOMATO DRESSING
CREAMY RASPBERRY DRESSING
"CAES-ARTS" SALAD DRESSING
CREOLE MUSTARD DRESSING
CREAMY HONEY MUSTARD DRESSING
SPICY TOMATO DRESSING

Thousand Island Dressing

*Zest of 2 Fresh Lemons — minced or 1 teaspoon dry
1 Small Carrot — peeled and minced (about ¼ cup)
1 teaspoon Oregano
3 Tablespoons White Vinegar
3 Tablespoons Water
3 teaspoons Sugar
¾ Cup Non-Fat Yogurt
¼ Cup Ketchup (preferably low calorie/low salt)
2 teaspoons Dry Parsley
1 Tablespoon Olive Oil (optional)

Put zest, carrots, oregano, vinegar, water and sugar in a saucepan and bring to a boil. Continue boiling until almost all the liquid is gone. Place this mixture in a medium bowl and add yogurt, ketchup and parsley and optional olive oil. Mix until well-blended and chill for 1-2 hours before serving.
YIELDS 1 CUP

A lemon zester is available at most gourmet stores. It is an inexpensive, but worthwhile tool for your kitchen.

NUTRITIONAL ANALYSIS
Per 1 Tbsp. Portion

Calories	13	Protein	1 gm
Fat	less than 1 gm	Carbohydrate	3 gm
Sodium	36 mg	Cholesterol	less than 1 mg

Sweet and Sour Tomato Dressing

1 6 oz. Can Tomato Paste
½ Cup Plus 2 Tablespoons White Vinegar
½ Cup Water
¼ Cup Molasses
¼ teaspoon White Pepper
¼ teaspoon Ground Coriander

Put all ingredients in a saucepan and with a whisk, blend until smooth. Bring mixture to a boil, stirring constantly. Reduce heat and simmer for 2 minutes. Chill for at least 1-2 hours before serving.
YIELDS ABOUT 1 CUP

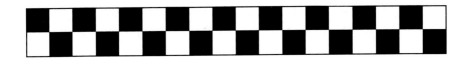

NUTRITIONAL ANALYSIS
Per 1 Tbsp. Portion

Calories	21	Protein	1 gm
Fat	less than 1 gm	Carbohydrate	5 gm
Sodium	89 mg	Cholesterol	0 mg

Creamy Raspberry Dressing

⅓ Cup Raspberry Vinegar
⅓ Cup Water
½ Cup Low-Fat Cottage Cheese
2 Tablespoons Pure Fruit Seedless Raspberry Jelly
1 Small Clove Garlic — minced
1 Small Onion — Chopped
  Juice of 1 Lemon
1 teaspoon Worcestershire Sauce
1 teaspoon Prepared Mustard (Dijon type preferably)
½ teaspoon Oregano
½ teaspoon Basil

Place all ingredients in a blender and blend until smooth.
YIELDS 1¼ CUPS

Note: Raspberry vinegar is available in most grocery stores or gourmet shops.

NUTRITIONAL ANALYSIS
Per 1 Tbsp. Portion

Calories	11	Protein	1 gm
Fat	less than 1 gm	Carbohydrate	2 gm
Sodium	34 mg	Cholesterol	less than 1 mg

"Caes-Art's" Dressing
or
Chef Arthur's Caesar Dressing

1 Cup Low-Fat Cottage Cheese
¼ Cup No Cholesterol, Reduced Calorie Mayonnaise
3 teaspoons Anchovy Paste
2 Cloves Garlic — crushed or minced
1 teaspoon Dry Mustard Powder
2 teaspoons White Vinegar
2 Tablespoons Water
¼ teaspoon Black Pepper
  Pinch of Cayenne Red Pepper

   Place all above ingredients in a processor and process until velvety smooth.
YIELDS 1¼ CUPS

NUTRITIONAL ANALYSIS
Per 1 Tbsp. Portion

Calories	21	Protein	2 gm
Fat	1 gm	Carbohydrate	less than 1 gm
Sodium	95 mg	Cholesterol	less than 1 mg

NOTE: High in fat, but great on occasion. To reduce fat, omit mayo.

Creole Mustard Dressing

½ Cup Low-Fat Cottage Cheese
2 Tablespoons Vegetable Oil (optional)
3 Tablespoons White Vinegar
2 Tablespoons + 1 teaspoon Creole Mustard or Dijon Type
1 Clove Garlic — minced
2 Tablespoons Water
1 teaspoon Dill
½ teaspoon Oregano
  Touch of Black Pepper
  Pinch of Cayenne Pepper

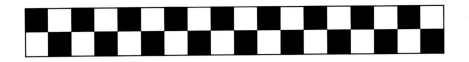

Combine cottage cheese, vegetable oil, vinegar, mustard, garlic and water in a blender. Process until smooth. Pour into large bowl and add dill, oregano, black pepper and cayenne pepper. Combine with a whisk until well-blended.
YIELDS ABOUT 1 CUP

NUTRITIONAL ANALYSIS
Per 1 Tbsp. Portion

Calories	9	Protein	less than 1 gm
Fat	less than 1 gm	Carbohydrate	less than 1 gm
Sodium	1 mg	Cholesterol	less than 1 mg

Creamy Honey Mustard Dressing

1 Cup Low-Fat Cottage Cheese
2 Tablespoons Dijon Mustard
2 Tablespoons Honey
1 Tablespoon Parsley (dry will do)
2 teaspoons White Vinegar
  Touch of Black Pepper
1 Tablespoon Water

Place all ingredients in a processor or blender and process until velvety smooth.
YIELDS 1¼ CUPS

NUTRITIONAL ANALYSIS
Per 1 Tbsp. Portion

Calories	16	Protein	1 gm
Fat	less than 1 gm	Carbohydrate	2 gm
Sodium	91 mg	Cholesterol	less than 1 mg

Spicy Tomato Dressing

¼ Cup Tomato Paste
½ Cup Water
2 Tablespoons Sugar
½ Cup White Vinegar
1 Tablespoon Creole Mustard or Dijon Style
1 Tablespoon Cornstarch
¼ teaspoon Black Pepper
   Cayenne Red Pepper to Taste (about ⅛ teaspoon or more)

    Combine all above ingredients in a saucepan and blend together with a whisk until smooth. Over high heat, bring to a boil, stirring constantly. Reduce heat to low and simmer 1 minute. Chill for at least 1-2 hours before serving.
YIELDS 1 CUP

NUTRITIONAL ANALYSIS
Per 1 Tbsp. Portion

Calories	13	Protein	less than 1 gm
Fat	less than 1 gm	Carbohydrate	3 gm
Sodium	61 mg	Cholesterol	0 mg

SAUCES

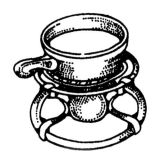

JAMAICAN BAY SAUCE
YOGURT AND CUCUMBER SAUCE
ORANGE DILL SAUCE
QUICK AND ZESTY TOMATO SAUCE

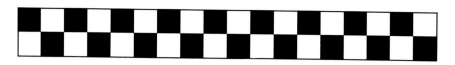

Jamaican Bay Sauce

1 Green Bell Pepper — chopped
1 Large Onion — chopped
1 Large Tomato — chopped
1 Fresh Jalapeno Pepper — finely chopped
3 Cloves Garlic — minced
¼ Cup Lime Juice
2 Tablespoons Fresh Ground Ginger
2 Tablespoons Lite Soy Sauce
1 Tablespoon Molasses
1 Tablespoon Mustard
¼ teaspoon Cinnamon
1 Cup Sherry
2 Tablespoons Cornstarch

Combine all ingredients except last two (sherry and cornstarch) in a saucepan. Bring to a boil, reduce heat to medium and cook for 3 minutes. In a separate dish mix sherry and cornstarch together until smooth and pour into simmering mixture. Bring to a boil once again, stirring constantly and remove from heat. This sauce is a great spicy seasoning for chicken, pork and fish. Serve it hot or cold.
YIELDS 2½ CUPS

NUTRITIONAL ANALYSIS
Per 1 Tbsp. Portion

Calories	8	Protein	less than 1 gm
Fat	less than 1 gm	Carbohydrate	2 gm
Sodium	37 mg	Cholesterol	0 mg

Yogurt and Cucumber Sauce

1 Cucumber (about ½ pound) — peeled, seeded and chopped
½ Cup Non-Fat Yogurt
1 teaspoon Chopped Fresh Mint (dry will do)

Combine all ingredients in a large bowl and mix well.
YIELDS 1¼ CUPS

NUTRITIONAL ANALYSIS
Per Recipe

Calories	98	Protein	7 gm
Fat	2 gm	Carbohydrate	14 gm
Sodium	91 mg	Cholesterol	7 mg

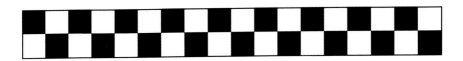

Orange Dill Sauce

2 Tablespoons Orange Juice Concentrate
1 Cup Non-Fat Yogurt
1 teaspoon Fresh Chopped Dill (dry will do)
1 Tablespoon Cornstarch

Place all ingredients in saucepan. Whisking constantly, bring to a boil over medium heat. Serve. Great on chicken, fish, pork, veal and soft shell crabs.
YIELDS 1 CUP

NUTRITIONAL ANALYSIS
Per 1 Tbsp. Portion

Calories	14	Protein	1 gm
Fat	less than 1 gm	Carbohydrate	3 gm
Sodium	11 mg	Cholesterol	less than 1 mg

Quick and Zesty Tomato Sauce

1 28 oz. Can Crushed Tomatoes
1 6 oz. Can Tomato Paste
1 Cup Water
½ Cup Dry White Wine or Water
1 Tablespoon White Vinegar
2 teaspoons Sugar
2 Cloves Garlic — minced
2 teaspoons Italian Seasoning
   Pinch of Cayenne Pepper (optional)

Place all above ingredients in an 8-quart dutch oven. Bring to a boil, reduce heat and simmer 20 minutes, stirring occasionally.
YIELDS 1 QUART

NUTRITIONAL ANALYSIS
Per Portion

Calories	111	Protein	5 gm
Fat	2 gm	Carbohydrate	22 gm
Sodium	744 mg	Cholesterol	2 mg

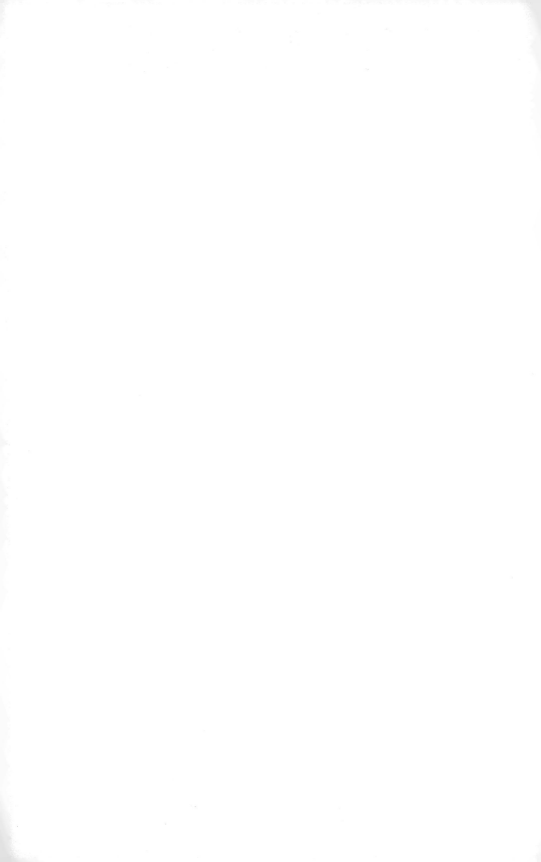

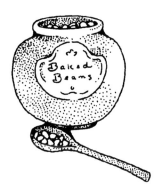

BEANS

HONEY BAKED BEANS
TWO BEAN OR NOT TO BEAN MARINADE
LENTIL STEW
PABLO'S BEAN AND CORN BAKE
KIDNEY BEANS AND RICE
BEANS AU MINT

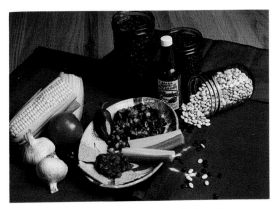

Pablo's Bean & Corn Bake — Salsa Picante

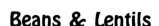

Beans & Lentils

Beans and lentils are great for you. It's that simple. For centuries, cultures around the world have lived on beans. They are high in protein and fiber, both vital to our good health.

It's been said that beans can stabilize blood sugar and they are credited with assisting in lowering cholesterol levels.

If you've tried dry beans before and don't care for them, try canned beans. As long as you rinse the canned version in a strainer under running water, they will provide the same benefits as home-cooked beans.

Total cooking time for beans varies, depending on the kind of bean. Your best bet is to follow package instructions, and don't forget to omit the salt. As a general rule, one cup of dry beans will provide two cups of cooked beans. Pretty great math, isn't it?

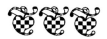

Honey Baked Beans

3 Cups Cooked Pinto Beans or 2, 15 oz. Cans Pinto Beans — rinsed
   under cold water and drained
1 Medium Onion — grated
1 Clove Garlic — minced
2 Tablespoons Tomato Paste
2 Tablespoons White Vinegar
2 Tablespoons Honey
1 Cup Water
1 Tablespoon Flour
   Pinch of Ground Cloves, Pinch of Allspice

Preheat oven to 375 degrees. Place all ingredients except beans in a large bowl and mix together until well-blended. Place the beans in a 2-quart baking dish, add sauce and mix well into beans. Place baking dish in oven and bake for 30 to 35 minutes.
SERVES 6

NUTRITIONAL ANALYSIS
Per Portion

Calories	154	Protein	8 gm
Fat	less than 1 gm	Carbohydrate	31 gm
Sodium	46 mg	Cholesterol	0 mg

Two Bean or Not to Bean Marinade

2 15 oz. Cans of Beans — 1 each of kidney, black, pinto, or
   great northern — rinsed under cold water and drained
1 Cup White Vinegar
1 Small Onion — chopped
1 Tablespoon Vegetable Oil
2 teaspoons Fresh Chopped Parsley (dry will do)
1 teaspoon Oregano
½ teaspoon Basil
2 teaspoons Sugar
4 Drops Hot Sauce (optional)

Place all ingredients in a medium bowl, mix well and allow to marinate in refrigerator for at least 1 hour.
SERVES 6

NUTRITIONAL ANALYSIS
Per Portion

Calories	128	Protein	7 gm
Fat	3 gm	Carbohydrate	19 gm
Sodium	214 mg	Cholesterol	0 mg

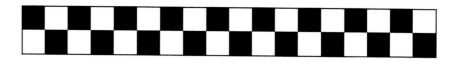

Lentil Stew

2 Cups Dried Lentils
3 Cups Vegetable Bouillon
1 Medium Onion — chopped
1 Stalk Celery — chopped
2 Cloves Garlic — minced
4 Potatoes — washed and cut into 1 inch cubes
1 Medium Tomato — chopped
½ teaspoon Oregano
2 Cups Skim Milk
  Juice of ½ Lemon

Wash lentils and place in an 8-quart dutch oven with vegetable bouillon, onion, celery and garlic. Bring this to a boil. Reduce heat and simmer for 15 minutes. Add remaining ingredients. Increase heat and bring to boil, uncovered. Reduce heat and simmer, stirring occasionally for another 15 to 20 minutes or until potatoes are tender.
YIELDS 8, 1-CUP SERVINGS

NUTRITIONAL ANALYSIS
Per 1 Cup Portion

Calories	240	Protein	17 gm
Fat	less than 1 gm	Carbohydrate	43 gm
Sodium	350 mg	Cholesterol	1 mg

Pablo's Bean and Corn Bake

1 Cup Cooked Corn (canned or frozen will do)
1 15 oz. Can Black Beans — rinsed under cold water and drained
1 4 oz. Jar Chopped Pimiento — rinsed under cold water and drained
1 Medium Onion — chopped
2 Cloves Garlic — minced
3 Tablespoons White Vinegar
2 Tablespoons Brown Sugar
1 8 oz. Can Tomato Sauce (no salt added)
1 Tablespoon Flour
2 teaspoons Chili Powder
¼ teaspoon Cumin
  Pinch of Cayenne Red Pepper

Preheat oven to 375 degrees. Place all ingredients except beans and corn in a large bowl. Mix together until well-blended. Mix beans and corn together in a 2-quart baking dish. Pour sauce over beans and corn and

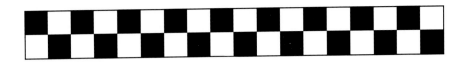

stir well. Place uncovered baking dish in preheated oven and bake for 40 to 45 minutes.
SERVES 6

NUTRITIONAL ANALYSIS
Per Portion

Calories	137	Protein	6 gm
Fat	less than 1 gm	Carbohydrate	28 gm
Sodium	296 mg	Cholesterol	0 mg

Kidney Beans and Rice

2 Cups Cooked Rice (follow package directions, but omit salt and butter)
2 Cups Cooked Kidney Beans or 1, 15 oz. Can of Kidney Beans —
    rinsed under cold water and drained
1 8 oz. Can Tomato Sauce (no salt added)
½ Cup Water
1 Medium Onion — chopped
1 Green Bell Pepper — chopped
1 Clove Garlic — minced
1 Tablespoon White Vinegar
    Pinch of Oregano
1 Bay Leaf
½ teaspoon Paprika
    Touch of Black Pepper

Prepare rice, set aside and keep warm. Put tomato sauce, water, onion, bell pepper, garlic, vinegar, oregano, bay leaf, paprika, black pepper and cayenne pepper in a saucepan and bring to a boil. Reduce heat and simmer uncovered for 10 minutes. Remove bay leaf and add beans. Simmer for another 5 minutes. Pour over warm, cooked rice and serve.
SERVES 4

NUTRITIONAL ANALYSIS
Per Portion

Calories	279	Protein	12 gm
Fat	1 gm	Carbohydrate	56 gm
Sodium	17 mg	Cholesterol	0 mg

Beans au Mint

1 19 oz. Can Canellini Beans or 15 oz. can Great Northern Beans
   rinsed under cold water and drained
1 Medium Carrot — finely shredded
¼ Cup Red Onion — chopped
¼ Cup White Vinegar
¼ Cup Water
   Juice of 1 Lemon
1 teaspoon Vegetable Oil
1 teaspoon Sugar
1 Tablespoon Fresh Chopped Parsley (dry will do)
1 Tablespoon Fresh Chopped Mint (dry will do)
   Touch of Black Pepper

   Place all ingredients in a medium bowl, mix well and allow to
marinate in refrigerator for 1 hour before serving.
SERVES 6

NUTRITIONAL ANALYSIS
Per Portion

Calories	84	Protein	5 gm
Fat	1 gm	Carbohydrate	14 gm
Sodium	116 mg	Cholesterol	0 mg

RICE DISHES

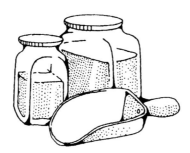

TOMATO RICE
DIRTY RICE
CURRIED RICE
LEMON RICE
SPINACH RICE

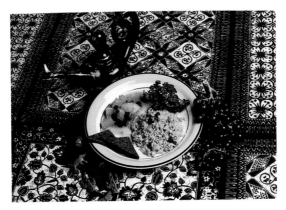

Curried Rice & Tropical Fruit Chutney

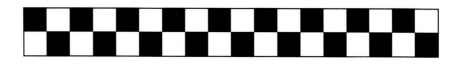

Rice

Rice is an excellent source of vitamins and nutrients. It's not fattening when it's eaten in place of a high-protein dish rather than a side dish with high protein. And if you don't drown it in butter it doesn't contain cholesterol.

Like most grain products, there is quite a variety of ways to prepare and serve rice. You can choose from brown rice, white rice, as well as the long and short grain versions.

My recipes in this book are prepared with long-grain rices because that's what is most commonly found in home pantries. However, I suggest you try brown rice because of its high fiber content. It takes longer to cook so adjust the cooking time according to package and recipe directions. Short grain rice serves well in puddings.

And we can't forget wild rice, which really isn't rice, but a seed. Once scarce, it's now easily available in most grocery stores. It can be prepared according to package directions.

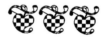

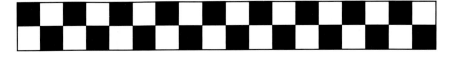

Tomato Rice

1 Medium Tomato — chopped
1 Small Onion — chopped
1 teaspoon Fresh Chopped Parsley (dry will do)
1 8 oz. Can Tomato Sauce (no salt added)
1 Cup Water
¼ teaspoon Black Pepper
1 Cup Dry Rice

Place all ingredients except rice in a saucepan and bring to a boil. Add rice and bring to a second boil. Reduce heat, cover and simmer for about 15 minutes or until rice is tender and liquid is absorbed.
SERVES 5

NUTRITIONAL ANALYSIS
Per Portion

Calories	159	Protein	4 gm
Fat	less than 1 gm	Carbohydrate	35 gm
Sodium	14 mg	Cholesterol	0 mg

Dirty Rice

1 Small Onion — chopped
1 Small Green Bell Pepper — chopped
1 Stalk Celery — chopped
2 Cloves Garlic — minced
1 teaspoon Paprika
½ teaspoon Dry Mustard
½ teaspoon Oregano
¼ teaspoon Basil
   Pinch of Cayenne Red Pepper
   Touch of Black Pepper
2 Cups Water
1 Cup Dry Rice

Place all ingredients except rice in a saucepan and bring to a boil. Add rice, bring to a second boil. Reduce heat, cover and simmer for about 15 minutes or until rice is tender and liquid is absorbed.
YIELDS 6 SERVINGS

NUTRITIONAL ANALYSIS
Per Portion

Calories	122	Protein	3 gm
Fat	less than 1 gm	Carbohydrate	27 gm
Sodium	8 mg	Cholesterol	0 mg

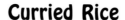

Curried Rice

¼ Cup Raisins
1 Clove Garlic — minced
½ teaspoon Onion Powder
2 teaspoons Curry Powder
1 teaspoon Cinnamon
2 Cups Chicken Bouillon (low-fat, low-sodium)
1 Cup Dry Rice

Place all ingredients except rice in a sauce pan and bring to a boil. Add rice and bring to second boil. Reduce heat, cover and simmer for about 15 minutes or until rice is tender and liquid is absorbed. Serve.
YIELDS 6 SERVINGS

NUTRITIONAL ANALYSIS
Per Portion

Calories	258	Protein	5 gm
Fat	1 gm	Carbohydrate	56 gm
Sodium	22 mg	Cholesterol	0 mg

Lemon Rice

2 Cups Chicken Broth (low-fat, low-sodium)
1 Tablespoon Fresh Chopped Parsley (dry will do)
3 Tablespoons Lemon Juice
  Pinch of Nutmeg
  Touch of Black Pepper
1 Cup Dry Rice

Place all ingredients except rice in a saucepan and bring to a boil. Add rice and bring to a second boil. Reduce heat, cover and simmer for 15 minutes or until rice is tender and liquid is absorbed.
SERVES 6

NUTRITIONAL ANALYSIS
Per Portion

Calories	125	Protein	3 gm
Fat	less than 1 gm	Carbohydrate	26 gm
Sodium	21 mg	Cholesterol	0 mg

Spinach Rice

1 10 oz. Package Frozen Chopped Spinach — thawed and drained
1 Medium Onion — chopped
1½ Cups Water
2 teaspoons Dill
⅔ Cup Dry Rice
3 teaspoons White Vinegar

Place thawed spinach, onion, water and dill in a saucepan. Bring to a boil and add rice. Bring to a second boil, reduce heat, cover and simmer for about 15 minutes or until rice is tender and liquid is absorbed. Add the vinegar, mix well and serve.
SERVES 4

NUTRITIONAL ANALYSIS
Per Portion

Calories	139	Protein	5 gm
Fat	less than 1 gm	Carbohydrate	30 gm
Sodium	55 mg	Cholesterol	0 mg

PASTA

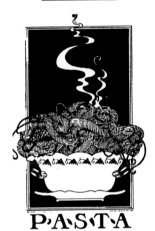

P·A·S·T·A

PASTA ITALIANO
PASTA "ART" FREDO WITH BROCCOLI
GARLIC PASTA SPINACI
EGGPLANT ATHENA ZITI
PASTA WITH FRESH TOMATO AND BASIL
PASTUNA

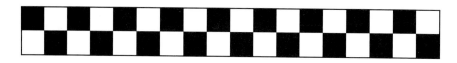

Pasta Italiano

12 Ounces Dry Pasta — spaghetti, elbows, vermicelli, etc. — your
  choice of shape
1 28 oz. Can Crushed Tomatoes
1 6 oz. Can Tomato Paste
1 Cup Water
½ Cup Dry Wine or Water
1 Tablespoon White Vinegar
2 teaspoons Sugar
2 Cloves Garlic — minced
2 Tablespoons Italian Spice
  Pinch of Cayenne Red Pepper (optional)
  Touch of Black Pepper
2 Tablespoons Grated Sap Sago Cheese (optional)

Prepare pasta according to package directions omitting salt. Drain
and keep hot. Place remaining ingredients except Sap Sago cheese in an
8-quart dutch oven. Mix until well-blended. Bring to boil, reduce heat and
simmer for 20 minutes, stirring occasionally. Keep sauce hot. Place cooked
pasta on serving platter and pour 2 cups of prepared tomato sauce over
pasta. Sprinkle grated Sap Sago cheese on top and serve.
SERVES 4
SAUCE YIELDS 1 QUART

Note: This is a very simple quick tomato sauce. It's good not only
for pasta but also for any dish requiring tomato sauce.

NUTRITIONAL ANALYSIS
Per Portion

Calories	371	Protein	13 gm
Fat	2 gm	Carbohydrate	74 gm
Sodium	378 mg	Cholesterol	1 mg

Pasta "ART" Fredo with Broccoli

12 Ounces Dry Pasta—linguini, spaghetti, vermicelli or your
  choice of shape
1¼ Cups Skim Milk
¼ Cup Low-Fat Ricotta Cheese
2 teaspoons Vegetable Oil
2 Tablespoons Flour
  Pinch of White Pepper
  Pinch of Nutmeg
3 Cups Broccoli Florets — steamed crisp
  Juice of ½ Lemon
2 Tablespoons Grated Sap Sago Cheese (optional)

Prepare pasta according to package directions, omitting salt. Drain
and keep hot. Pour skim milk, ricotta cheese, oil, flour, pepper and nutmeg
into a saucepan. Stirring constantly over high heat, bring to a boil. Reduce
heat to low and simmer for 7 minutes, stirring occasionally. Put pasta into
a large bowl and add sauce, broccoli and lemon juice. Toss until well
mixed. Serve with fresh grated Sap Sago cheese on top.
SERVES 4

NUTRITIONAL ANALYSIS
Per Portion

Calories	434	Protein	20 gm
Fat	5 gm	Carbohydrate	77 gm
Sodium	140 mg	Cholesterol	5 mg

Garlic Pasta Spinaci

12 Ounces Dry Pasta — elbows, ziti, vermicelli, etc.
1½ Cups Chicken Stock (low-fat, low-sodium)
2 Tablespoons Flour
1 10 oz. Package Frozen Chopped Spinach
4 Cloves Garlic — minced
2 teaspoons Vegetable Oil
   Touch of Black Pepper
   Pinch of Cayenne Red Pepper
   Juice of ½ Lemon
2 Tablespoons Grated Sap Sago Cheese (optional)

   Prepare pasta according to package directions omitting salt. Drain and keep hot. Pour chicken stock into saucepan and add flour. Stir until smooth. Over high heat, bring to a boil, reduce heat to low and simmer 7 minutes, stirring occasionally. While stock is cooking put oil in a small (6 inch), non-stick skillet over medium heat and add garlic. Stirring with a wooden spoon, cook garlic for 1 minute. Do not let garlic get brown or burn as this makes it very bitter. Remove cooked garlic from pan and set aside. Prepare spinach according to package directions. Drain in a strainer and squeeze almost dry. Place cooked pasta in a large bowl and add cooked chicken stock, drained spinach, garlic and the rest of the ingredients except Sap Sago cheese. Toss until well-mixed, sprinkle grated Sap Sago cheese on top and serve.
SERVES 4

NUTRITIONAL ANALYSIS
Per Portion

Calories	401	Protein	15 gm
Fat	5 gm	Carbohydrate	73 gm
Sodium	116 mg	Cholesterol	2 mg

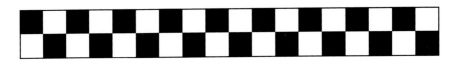

Eggplant Athena Ziti

12 Ounces Dry Pasta — ziti, elbows, shells or your choice of shape
1 Medium Eggplant (1 pound) — cut off stem but do not peel —
   chop into ¼ inch pieces
1 Small Onion — grated
18 Ounces Beef Stock (low-fat, low-sodium)
1 8 oz. Can Tomato Sauce (no salt added)
½ Cup Fresh chopped Parsley (dry will do)
2 Cloves Garlic — minced
¼ teaspoon Allspice
   Touch of Black Pepper
   Pinch of Cayenne Red Pepper (optional)
¼ Cup Port Wine or ¼ Cup Water Plus 2 teaspoons Sugar
¼ Cup Ricotta Cheese, low-fat
2 Tablespoons Flour
2 Tablespoons Grated Sap Sago Cheese (optional)

Prepare pasta according to package directions omitting salt, drain and keep hot. Place eggplant, onion, beef stock, tomato sauce, parsley, garlic, allspice and red and black pepper in an 8-quart dutch oven. Bring to boil, reduce heat and simmer for 20 minutes stirring occasionally. Meanwhile put wine, ricotta cheese and flour in a blender and blend until smooth. When eggplant sauce has simmered for 20 minutes add the ricotta cheese mixture and blend in well with a wooden spoon. Once again bring to a boil, reduce heat and simmer for 7 more minutes stirring occasionally. Place pasta into a large bowl and add sauce. Toss until well-mixed. Sprinkle grated Sap Sago cheese on top and serve.
SERVES 4

NUTRITIONAL ANALYSIS
Per Portion

Calories	411	Protein	16 gm
Fat	3 gm	Carbohydrate	82 gm
Sodium	44 mg	Cholesterol	1 mg

Pasta with Fresh Tomato and Basil

12 Ounces Dry Pasta — spaghetti, linguini, elbows or
   your choice of shape
1½ Cups Chicken Stock (low-fat, low sodium)
2 Tablespoons Flour
2 Fresh Ripe Tomatoes — chopped
3 teaspoons Fresh Chopped Basil or 2 teaspoons dry
   Touch of Black Pepper
   Pinch Cayenne Red Pepper
   Juice ½ Lemon
2 Tablespoons Grated Sap Sago Cheese (optional)

      Prepare pasta according to package directions omitting salt. Drain
and keep hot. Pour chicken stock into sauce pot and add flour. Stir until
smooth. Over high heat, bring to boil. Reduce heat to low and simmer
7 minutes stirring occasionally. While stock is cooking put oil in a small
(6 inch) non-stick skillet over medium heat. Add garlic and cook it for
1 minute stirring with a wooden spoon. Do not let garlic get brown or
burn as this makes it very bitter. Remove from pan and set aside. Place
cooked pasta in a large bowl and add cooked chicken stock, tomatoes,
garlic and the rest of the ingredients except Sap Sago cheese. Toss until
well-mixed. Sprinkle grated Sap Sago cheese on top and serve.
SERVES 4

NUTRITIONAL ANALYSIS
Per Portion

Calories	373	Protein	13 gm
Fat	3 gm	Carbohydrate	72 gm
Sodium	68 mg	Cholesterol	2 mg

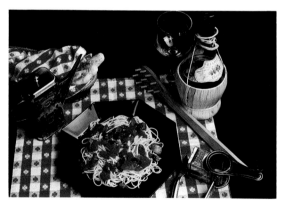

Tomato & Basil Pasta

Pastuna

12 Ounces Dry Pasta — medium shells, elbows, bows or
  your choice of shape
1 15 oz. Can Stewed Tomatoes — no salt added
1 6 oz. Can Water Packed Tuna — rinsed and drained
1 Medium Zucchini (about ½ pound) — shredded
1 8 oz. Can Tomato Sauce — no salt added
3 Tablespoons Tomato Paste
¼ Cup White Vinegar
¼ Cup Dry Wine
2 Cloves Garlic — minced
1 teaspoon Oregano
½ teaspoon Basil
    Pinch of Rosemary
    Touch of Black Pepper
    Pinch of Cayenne Red Pepper
2 Tablespoons Grated Sap Sago Cheese (optional)

Prepare pasta according to package directions omitting salt. Drain
and keep hot. Place all ingredients except cooked pasta and Sap Sago
cheese in saucepan and bring to a boil. Reduce heat and simmer for
20 minutes, stirring occasionally. Put cooked pasta into a large bowl and
add sauce. Toss until well-mixed. Sprinkle Sap Sago cheese on top and
serve.
SERVES 4

NUTRITIONAL ANALYSIS
Per Portion

Calories	447	Protein	26 gm
Fat	2 gm	Carbohydrate	81 gm
Sodium	307 mg	Cholesterol	17 mg

VEGETABLE DISHES

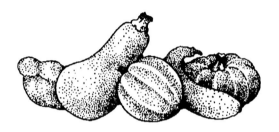

BAKED EGGPLANT
STUFFED TOMATOES NEW DELHI
VEGETABLE & BEAN HASH
POT OF VEGETABLES
STUFFED ZUCCHINI WITH TOMATO SAUCE
CAJUN VEGETABLE ETOUFFEE

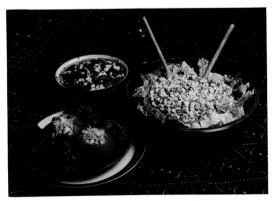

Calico Salad, Stuffed Tomatoes New Delhi &
Two Bean or Not to Bean Marinade

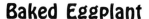

Baked Eggplant

1 Large Eggplant (about ½ pound) — cut into 1 inch cubes
1½ Cups Cooked Bulgur Wheat (follow package directions, but omit salt)
1 Medium Onion — chopped
1 Medium Green Bell Pepper — chopped
1 Medium Tomato — chopped
¼ Cup Tomato Paste
1 teaspoon Oregano
½ teaspoon Paprika
½ teaspoon Allspice or Apple Pie Spice
   Touch of Black Pepper

     Preheat Oven to 350 degrees.
     Cook cubed eggplant in boiling water for 10 minutes, drain and set aside. Prepare bulgur wheat. Combine all above remaining ingredients except eggplant in a large bowl. Now add cooked eggplant and gently toss into mixture. Spoon well-blended mixture into a lightly oiled (¼ tsp. vegetable oil) casserole dish. Place in a preheated 350 degree oven for 30 minutes.
     Serve with Yogurt and Cucumber Sauce. (See Sauces)
YIELDS 6 SERVINGS

NUTRITIONAL ANALYSIS
Per Portion

Calories	92	Protein	4 gm
Fat	less than 1 gm	Carbohydrate	21 gm
Sodium	95 mg	Cholesterol	0 mg

Stuffed Tomatoes New Delhi

1½ Cups Cooked Rice (follow package directions but omit salt and butter)
6 Large Tomatoes
1 15 oz. Can Great Northern Beans or Navy Beans — rinsed and drained
1 Tablespoon Honey
1 teaspoon Curry
1 Small Onion — chopped
1 Medium Banana — peeled, split lengthwise and cut into ½ inch pieces
1 Apple — cored and chopped
2 Cloves Garlic — minced
2 Tablespoons Tomato Paste
1 Tablespoon Honey
1 teaspoon Curry

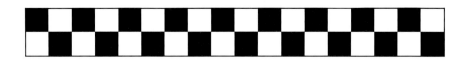

1 teaspoon Allspice
¼ teaspoon Cayenne Pepper
  Non-stick Cooking Spray for Baking Dish

    Preheat oven to 375 degrees.
    Prepare rice according to package directions omitting salt and butter. Cut a slice off tops of tomatoes and scoop out pulp. Chop removed pulp and put in large bowl with the remaining ingredients except non-stick cooking spray. Stir to blend ingredients well. Spoon into scooped out tomatoes. Lightly spray a 2-quart baking dish or pan with non-stick cooking spray. Put stuffed tomatoes in baking dish and bake at 375 degrees for 20 minutes or until tomatoes are tender.
SERVES 6

NUTRITIONAL ANALYSIS
Per Portion

Calories	220	Protein	8 gm
Fat	1 gm	Carbohydrate	47 gm
Sodium	60 mg	Cholesterol	0 mg

Vegetable & Bean Hash

1 Pound Broccoli — chopped into 1 inch pieces
2 Medium Onions — diced into ½ inch pieces
4 Tomatoes — diced into ½ inch pieces
3 Medium Zucchini — diced into ½ inch pieces
3 Cloves Garlic — minced
¼ Cup Sherry or Water
1 teaspoon Thyme
1 teaspoon Basil
  Touch of Black Pepper
1 15 oz. Can Whole Kernel Corn — rinsed and drained
1 15 oz. Can Butter Beans — rinsed and drained

    Combine all ingredients except corn and beans in an 8-quart dutch oven. Cook for 6 minutes, stirring occasionally. Stir in drained corn and beans and cook for 2 minutes more. Serve.
YIELDS 4-6 SERVINGS

NUTRITIONAL ANALYSIS
Per Portion

Calories	181	Protein	11 gm
Fat	2 gm	Carbohydrate	38 gm
Sodium	304 mg	Cholesterol	0 mg

Pot of Vegetables

4 Medium Potatoes — peeled and cut into wedges
4 Large Carrots — peeled, split in half, lengthwise and cut into
    2 inch pieces
8 Small Onions — peeled and cut in half
1 15 oz. Can Kernel Corn — rinsed and drained
½ Cup Sherry or Water
2 Tablespoons Lemon Juice
3 Tablespoons Parsley
   Touch of Black Pepper

    Preheat oven to 300 degrees.
    Wash and prepare all vegetables. Place vegetables in an 8-quart dutch oven with a tight fitting lid. Pour sherry and lemon juice over them, sprinkle parsley and pepper on top. Toss vegetables lightly to mix. Put cover on pot and place in preheated 300 degree oven for 2 hours.
SERVES 6

NUTRITIONAL ANALYSIS
Per Portion

Calories	160	Protein	4 gm
Fat	less than 1 gm	Carbohydrate	37 gm
Sodium	33 mg	Cholesterol	0 mg

Stuffed Zucchini with Tomato Sauce

1 Cup Cooked Rice (follow package directions, but omit salt and butter)
2 Medium Zucchini about ½ pound each
¼ teaspoon Vegetable Oil
1 Medium Onion — chopped
1 Stalk Celery — finely chopped
2 Tablespoons Water (or more if needed)
¼ Cup Bread Crumbs
¼ Cup Hoop Cheese (See Appetizers Section)
2 Egg Whites

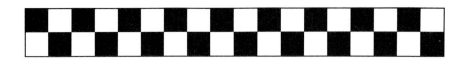

2 Tablespoons Tomato Paste
2 Tablespoons Chopped Parsley
1 teaspoon Thyme
  Touch of Black Pepper

Preheat oven to 350 degrees.

Prepare rice according to package directions omitting salt and butter. Set aside. Trim stems off zucchini, cut zucchini in half lengthwise and
scoop out pulp leaving about a ¼" wall around zucchini. (Use a melon
baller or teaspoon.) Chop zucchini pulp. Place zucchini pulp, onion, celery,
tomato and water in a 12", non-stick skillet and cook over medium-high
heat until almost all of the liquid is gone. Place this mixture in a large
bowl and add the remaining ingredients, mixing thoroughly. Spoon the
mixture into the hollowed zucchini halves and press in firmly. Place in
a lightly oiled baking dish, pour tomato sauce on top and bake for 30
minutes in a preheated 350 degree oven.
SERVES 4

Tomato Sauce:
½ Cup Tomato Paste
1 Cup Water
1 Clove Garlic — minced
Thoroughly mix all ingredients in a medium bowl.
YIELDS 1½ CUPS

NUTRITIONAL ANALYSIS
Per Portion

Calories	163	Protein	9 gm
Fat	1 gm	Carbohydrate	31 gm
Sodium	469 mg	Cholesterol	less than 1 mg

Cajun Vegetable Etouffee (A-Too-Fay)

4-5 Cups Fresh Vegetables Of Your Choice — cut into bitesize pieces — example: zucchini, yellow squash, onions, red and green bell peppers, carrots, green onions, mushrooms, etc.
2 Tablespoons Vegetable Oil for Roux
3 Tablespoons Flour for Roux
1 Medium Onion — chopped
1 Stalk Celery — chopped
1 Medium Green or Red Bell Pepper — chopped
2 Cloves Garlic — minced
1 teaspoon Italian Seasoning
1 teaspoon Paprika
¼ teaspoon Black Pepper
   Pinch of Cayenne Pepper (more or less to taste)
1½ Cups Vegetable Broth
2 Cups Cooked Rice — follow package directions, but omit salt and butter

Steam prepared vegetables that were cut into bitesize pieces until crisp tender or to desired doneness. Set aside. Place oil and flour in a large saute skillet and cook over medium heat stirring often until gold to dark brown. When roux reaches desired color, add chopped onion, chopped bell pepper, chopped celery, minced garlic, Italian seasoning, paprika, cayenne and black pepper. Saute until vegetables in roux are soft. Allow this to cool. When cool, add vegetable stock to roux mixture. Whisking constantly, bring to a boil over medium-high heat until well blended. Stir in steamed vegetables. To serve, mound ½ cup cooked rice on each plate and surround the rice with ¾ cup of vegetable etouffee per person.
SERVES 4

NUTRITIONAL ANALYSIS
Per Portion

Calories	270	Protein	6 gm
Fat	8 gm	Carbohydrate	45 gm
Sodium	333 mg	Cholesterol	0 mg

FISH DISHES

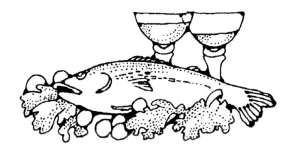

**SPICY FISH CREOLE
POACHED FISH
HONEY MUSTARD FISH WITH CURRY
FLOUNDER ROLLUPS
FISH AND ONIONS BARBADOS
FILET OF SOLE IN WHITE WINE SAUCE**

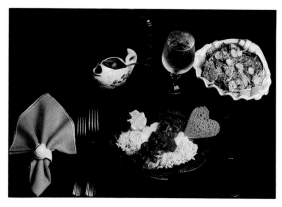

Spicy Fish Creole & Caes-Art's Salad

Meat Dishes

I consider fish, chicken, turkey, pork and beef all meat dishes. You can see by the nutritional analysis of each of the Fish Dishes, Poultry Dishes and Pork and Beef Dishes, that fish is the lowest in fat. However, this does not give you license to overindulge in fish. As a matter of fact, or should I say, as a matter of FAT, the optimum consumption of animal protein should not exceed 3 to 4 ounces of meat per day. How much is 3 to 4 ounces of meat, you ask? About the size of a deck of cards. Go easy on animal protein. Your innards will love you and so will your waistline.

Spicy Fish Creole

4 4 oz. Portions of Skinless White Non-Oily Fish Filets (cod, haddock, flounder, snapper, etc.) — rinsed and patted dry
2 Cups Cooked Rice (optional) (omit salt and butter)
1 Medium Onion — peeled and chopped
1 Medium Green Bell Pepper — seeded and chopped
2 Stalks Celery cut into ½ inch pieces
¼ Cup Water
1 Large Tomato, chopped
2 Cloves Garlic — minced
½ teaspoon Oregano
½ teaspoon Rosemary
1 teaspoon Paprika
⅛ teaspoon Cayenne Pepper
1 Tablespoon Worcestershire Sauce
1 Tablespoon Water
1 Tablespoon Cornstarch

To Cook Fish:
Follow Poached Fish recipe. Place cooked fish on serving platter and keep warm.

In a 12", non-stick skillet, combine onion, bell pepper, celery and water. Over high heat bring to a boil, reduce heat and simmer covered for 4 to 5 minutes or until vegetables are tender. Add tomatoes, garlic, oregano, rosemary, paprika and cayenne pepper to vegetable mixture and cook 4 to 5 minutes more. In a separate bowl whisk together until smooth worcestershire, water and cornstarch. Stir this mixture into the vegetable mixture and cook until thick and bubbly (about 2 minutes). Pour over fish and serve. (Serve with rice optional).
SERVES 4

NUTRITIONAL ANALYSIS
Per Portion

Calories	131	Protein	21 gm
Fat	1 gm	Carbohydrate	8 gm
Sodium	125 mg	Cholesterol	49 mg

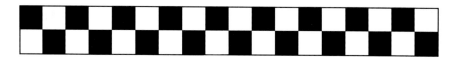

Poached Fish

4 4 oz. Portions of Skinless White Non-Oily Fish Filets (cod,
   haddock, flounder, snapper, etc.) — rinsed and patted dry
2 Lemon Slices
1 Bay Leaf
1 Slice Onion
3 Whole Cloves
3 Tablespoons White Vinegar
   Water — enough to cover fish

   Fill a 12″, non-stick skillet with enough water to cover the fish by
½ inch. Add all ingredients except fish. Bring to boil and reduce heat to
medium. Add fish filets and poach for 10 to 15 minutes. Fish is done when
center of filet is opaque in color. Carefully remove fish with spatula and
place on serving plates.
   Poached fish goes well with my Jamaican Bay Sauce or Cucumber
Yogurt Sauce. Be creative.
SERVES 4

NUTRITIONAL ANALYSIS
Per Portion

Calories	98	Protein	20 gm
Fat	less than 1 gm	Carbohydrate	2 gm
Sodium	62 mg	Cholesterol	49 mg

Honey Mustard Fish with Curry

4 4 oz. Portions of Skinless White Non-Oily Fish Filets (cod,
   haddock, flounder, snapper, etc.) — rinsed and patted dry
¼ teaspoon Vegetable Oil
2 Tablespoons Honey
2 teaspoons Prepared Mustard
1 Tablespoon Lemon Juice
1 teaspoon Curry Powder
   Touch of Cayenne Pepper

   Preheat oven to 350 degrees.
   Place fish filets in a lightly oiled baking dish. In a small bowl mix
the remaining ingredients and pour over the fish. Bake in a 350 degree
oven for 30 minutes or until fish flakes easily when separated with a fork.
SERVES 4

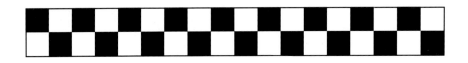

NUTRITIONAL ANALYSIS
Per Portion

Calories	130	Protein	21 gm
Fat	1 gm	Carbohydrate	10 gm
Sodium	96 mg	Cholesterol	49 mg

Flounder Rollups with Orange Dill Sauce

6 Flounder Filets without Skin
1 Pound Fresh Asparagus (frozen will do — 2 to 3
    spears per Fish Filet)
1 Cup White Wine or Water
1 Prepared Recipe Orange Dill Sauce (See Sauces)

In a 12″, non-stick skillet, simmer asparagus for 4 minutes in water. Remove asparagus from water and drain. On table, lay flounder filets skinned side down and place 2 to 3 asparagus spears on the large end of each filet so the spears visibly stick out on sides. From large end of the filet, roll the asparagus in the fish filet and place seam side down in a 12″, non-stick skillet. Pour cup of wine over fish rollups and simmer covered for 4 to 5 minutes. Remove fish very carefully with a slotted spoon to serving dish. Top with zesty Orange Dill Sauce already prepared. Serve.
SERVES 6

NUTRITIONAL ANALYSIS
Per Portion

Calories	184	Protein	32 gm
Fat	2 gm	Carbohydrate	10 gm
Sodium	148 mg	Cholesterol	69 mg

Fish and Onions Barbados

4 4 oz. Portions of Skinless White Non-Oily Fish Filets (cod,
   haddock, flounder, snapper, etc.) — rinsed and patted dry
2 Medium Onions — peeled and thinly sliced
8 Green Onions — chopped (green tops, too)
¼ Cup White Wine or Water
2 Tablespoons White Vinegar
2 teaspoons Sugar
   Pinch of Cayenne Pepper
   Water

To Cook Fish:
   Follow Poached Fish recipe. Place on serving platter and keep fish
warm.
   Place onions, green onions, wine, vinegar, sugar and cayenne
pepper in a 10″, non-stick skillet over medium to medium-high heat. Cook
onions for 10 minutes or until tender. Add water one tablespoon at a time
to onions if needed. When onions are tender, spoon over fish and serve.
SERVES 4

NOTE: A similar fish dish is served frequently in the Carribean Islands.
There they incorporate very hot Scotch Bonnet Peppers into the onions.
So if you like it hot add your favorite hot sauce or more cayenne pepper.

NUTRITIONAL ANALYSIS
Per Portion

Calories	124	Protein	21 gm
Fat	less than 1 gm	Carbohydrate	7 gm
Sodium	64 mg	Cholesterol	49 mg

Filet of Sole in White Wine

4 4 oz. Portions of Skinless Filets of Sole (cod, haddock, flounder,
   etc. may be used) — rinsed and patted dry
1 teaspoon Vegetable Oil
¼ Cup White Wine
   Juice of 1 Lemon
½ teaspoon Parsley (dry will do)
¼ teaspoon Tarragon
¼ teaspoon Rosemary
¼ teaspoon Thyme
   Touch of Pepper

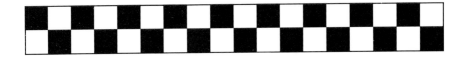

Preheat oven to 350 degrees.

Place fish filets in a lightly oiled baking dish. Combine remaining ingredients in a medium bowl and pour over fish. Bake at 350 degrees for 30 minutes.
SERVES 4

NUTRITIONAL ANALYSIS
Per Portion

Calories	119	Protein	21 gm
Fat	2.5 gm	Carbohydrate	2 gm
Sodium	93 mg	Cholesterol	54 mg

POULTRY DISHES

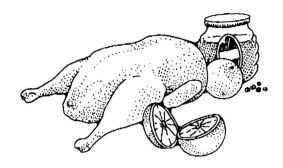

CRISPY OVEN-FRIED CHICKEN
CHICKEN MARSALA
TURKEY VEGGIE BURGERS
TANGY CHICKEN WITH TOMATO SAUCE
CHICKEN POT STEW
TURKEY DRUMS WITH APPLES AND HERBS
CHICKEN ETOUFFEE
MARINATED CHICKEN

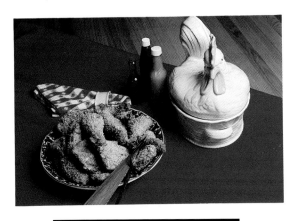

Crispy
Oven-Fried Chicken

Crispy Oven-Fried Chicken

1½-2 Pounds Chicken Legs — skin and fat removed
4 Large Shredded Wheat Biscuits — crushed
¼ Cup Bread Crumbs
1 Cup Non-Fat Yogurt
1 Tablespoon Lemon Juice
½ teaspoon Onion Powder
½ teaspoon Oregano
1 teaspoon Cornstarch
   Pinch of Cayenne Pepper

   Preheat oven to 375 degrees.
   In a large bowl blend together yogurt, lemon juice, onion powder, oregano, cornstarch and cayenne pepper. Dip skinless chicken into this mixture making sure that every piece is coated completely. In a shallow pan, mix bread crumbs and crushed shredded wheat biscuits thoroughly. Take chicken from yogurt mixture and place it in the crumb mixture covering all sides well. Fit 2 cake cooling racks on your baking sheet pan. Make sure you oil the racks if they are not non-stick. Place all of the coated chicken on the racks and bake in a preheated 375 degree oven for 55 to 60 minutes. Turn the chicken over once in the last 10 minutes of cooking time. Remove from oven onto serving dish and serve.
SERVES 4

NUTRITIONAL ANALYSIS
Per Portion

Calories	297	Protein	30 gm
Fat	5 gm	Carbohydrate	32 gm
Sodium	188 mg	Cholesterol	92 mg

Chicken Marsala

1 2.5 to 3 Pound Chicken — skin, backbone and all visible fat removed,
   cut into serving pieces
½ teaspoon Vegetable Oil
   Touch of Black Pepper
1 teaspoon Basil
2 8 oz. Cans Tomato Sauce — no salt added
1 Fresh Tomato — chopped
3 Cloves Garlic — minced or crushed
2 Tablespoons Fresh Parsley — chopped (dry will do)

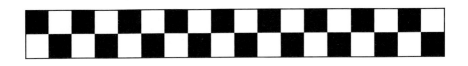

¾ Cup Marsala Wine
1 teaspoon Oregano
   Touch of Cayenne Pepper
2 Tablespoons Miller's Bran or Bread Crumbs

   Preheat oven to 350 degrees.
   Sprinkle chicken pieces generously with pepper and basil and place in a lightly oiled 12", non-stick skillet. Over medium heat, saute chicken until brown on all sides. While chicken is browning, put the rest of the ingredients in a bowl and mix thoroughly. Remove browned chicken from pan and place in a baking dish. Pour sauce on top of chicken and bake for 35-40 minutes in a 350 degree oven.
SERVES 2 to 3

NUTRITIONAL ANALYSIS
Per Portion

Calories	341	Protein	46 gm
Fat	7 gm	Carbohydrate	24 gm
Sodium	197 mg	Cholesterol	140 mg

Turkey Veggie Burgers

1 Pound Fresh Ground Turkey Breast
1 Pound Finely Shredded Vegetables (carrots, zucchini, onions, yellow squash, red and green bell peppers, etc.)
1 Tablespoon Worcestershire Sauce
½ teaspoon Italian Seasoning
1 Clove Garlic — minced
   Pinch of Cayenne Pepper
   Touch of Ground Black Pepper

   Mix all above ingredients together in a large bowl until evenly blended and smooth. Form into burger patties and cook over medium heat in a 12", non-stick skillet until done, about 4 to 5 minutes on each side.
MAKES 6 to 8 BURGERS

NUTRITIONAL ANALYSIS
Per 1 Each Portion

Calories	114	Protein	12 gm
Fat	5 gm	Carbohydrate	5 gm
Sodium	93 mg	Cholesterol	47 mg

A little high in fat; o.k. occasionally. To reduce fat, increase vegetables.

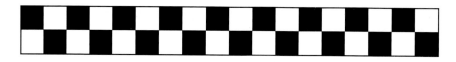

Tangy Chicken with Tomato Sauce

1 2.5 Pound Chicken — remove skin and all fat, cut into serving pieces
2 teaspoons Dried Tarragon
  Touch of Black Pepper
1 teaspoon Vegetable Oil for Saute
2 Tomatoes — coarsely chopped
1 8 oz. Can Tomato Sauce (no salt added)
½ Cup Red Wine Vinegar
3 Cloves Garlic — minced
1 teaspoon Dried Tarragon
1 Tablespoon Molasses

Preheat oven to 350 degrees.
Sprinkle tarragon and pepper on chicken pieces. Place chicken pieces in a lightly oiled 12", non-stick skillet with an oven-proof handle, and brown for 5 to 6 minutes on each side. Put the rest of the ingredients in a bowl and mix together. When chicken is browned, pour the mixture on top of the chicken in the skillet and place skillet in preheated 350 degree oven for 35 to 40 minutes.* Take skillet out of oven and place on burner over medium-high heat. Remove chicken pieces to serving dish. Cook remaining sauce until thick. Pour sauce over chicken and serve.
SERVES 4 *Remember the handle is very hot so use a potholder.

NUTRITIONAL ANALYSIS
Per Portion

Calories	228	Protein	31 gm
Fat	6 gm	Carbohydrate	13 gm
Sodium	129 mg	Cholesterol	95 mg

Chicken Pot Stew

1 2.5 Pound Chicken — remove skin and all fat, cut into serving pieces
4 Medium Potatoes — peeled and cut into wedges
3 Carrots (about 1 pound) — peeled, split in half and cut into
  2 inch lengths
4 Stalks Celery — cut into 2 inch lengths
4 Onions — peeled and quartered
4 Ounces Beer
2 Tablespoons Lemon Juice
1 Tablespoon Parsley (dry will do)
1 teaspoon Oregano
  Touch of Black Pepper

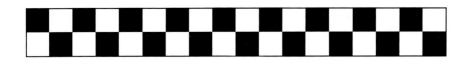

Preheat oven to 350 degrees.

Place chicken in bottom of an 8-quart dutch oven. Put all prepared vegetables on top of chicken. Pour beer and lemon juice over chicken and vegetables. Add parsley, oregano and pepper. Cover with tight lid and place in preheated 350 degree oven. Bake for 2 hours and serve.
SERVES 4 to 6

NUTRITIONAL ANALYSIS
Per Portion

Calories	348	Protein	34 gm
Fat	5 gm	Carbohydrate	43 gm
Sodium	188 mg	Cholesterol	96 mg

Turkey Drums with Apples and Herbs

2 Turkey Drumsticks — skin removed
　Touch of Pepper
¼ teaspoon Onion Powder
¼ teaspoon Garlic Powder
1 Apple — peeled, cored and chopped
¼ Cup Apple Juice
¼ Cup Lemon Juice
1 teaspoon Oregano
¼ teaspoon Tarragon
1 Tablespoon Flour
2 Slices Lemon per Drumstick
　Water

Preheat oven to 350 degrees.

Sprinkle drumsticks with pepper, onion powder and garlic powder. In a lightly oiled 12", non-stick skillet, brown drumsticks on all sides. In a saucepan put apples, apple juice, lemon juice, oregano, tarragon and flour. Bring to a boil, stirring constantly. Reduce heat to medium and simmer for 1 minute. Place turkey drums in a lightly oiled baking dish. Pour this mixture over them and place 2 lemon slices on top. Bake in a preheated 350 degree oven for 2½ to 3 hours, basting occasionally. Check liquid level and add a little water when necessary. Discard lemon slices. When done, the meat will be real tender. Remove meat from bone, place on serving platter. Pour sauce on top and serve.
SERVES 4

NUTRITIONAL ANALYSIS
Per Portion

Calories	227	Protein	32 gm
Fat	7 gm	Carbohydrate	10 gm
Sodium	127 mg	Cholesterol	115 mg

Chicken Etouffee (A-Too-Fay)

2 Tablespoons Vegetable Oil for Roux
3 Tablespoons Flour for Roux
1 Medium Onion — finely chopped
1 Medium Bell Pepper — finely chopped
1 Stalk Celery — finely chopped
2 Green Onions — finely chopped (green tops, too)
2 Cloves Garlic — minced
1 teaspoon Paprika
1 teaspoon Oregano
½ teaspoon Rosemary
¼ teaspoon Black Pepper
⅛ teaspoon Cayenne Pepper (more or less to taste)
1 Cup Chicken Broth (low sodium)
1 Pound Skinless, Boneless Chicken Breast — cut into 1 inch cubes
2 Cups Cooked Rice (follow package instructions, but omit salt)

To Prepare Roux:

Please Note: Cooked roux is very, very hot and it sticks to your skin like glue. Please be careful!
Pour oil into a 10", non-stick skillet and heat over medium high heat. When oil is very hot, reduce heat to low and add flour. Blend flour into oil with a wooden spoon until mixture is smooth. Adjust heat so mixture cooks making tiny bubbles (low to medium heat). Stirring often, it should take about 12 to 15 minutes for the mixture to become the desired dark golden brown color.

To Prepare Etouffee:

When roux reaches desired color, very carefully add onion, bell pepper, celery, green onions, garlic, paprika, oregano, rosemary, black pepper and cayenne pepper to the roux and saute until vegetables are soft (about 7 to 10 minutes). Set aside. In a medium saucepan over high heat, bring 1 cup of chicken broth to a boil. Reduce heat to low. Carefully add vegetable roux mixture to the broth. Turn heat to high once again. Whisking constantly, cook mixture until well-blended. Add chicken pieces, turn heat to low, cover pot and simmer for about 10 to 15 minutes or until chicken is cooked but tender. Stir occasionally.
To serve, mound ½ cup of cooked rice on each plate and surround the rice with ¾ cup of etouffee per person.
SERVES 4

NUTRITIONAL ANALYSIS
Per Portion

Calories	360	Protein	30 gm
Fat	9 gm	Carbohydrate	38 gm
Sodium	87 mg	Cholesterol	66 mg

Marinated Chicken

4 Chicken Breasts — all skin and visible fat removed
1 Tablespoon Vegetable Oil
  Juice of 3 lemons
2 Cloves Garlic — minced
1 teaspoon Dried Oregano
1 teaspoon Dried Basil
  Touch of Black Pepper

Preheat oven to 350 degrees.
Wash chicken and pat dry. Mix all above ingredients together in a glass baking dish. Put chicken in dish with marinade and refrigerate at least 2 hours. Remove chicken from marinade (reserve marinade) and place in a 12", non-stick skillet that has a heatproof handle. Brown chicken over medium-high heat for about 2½ minutes on each side. When chicken is brown, pour the remaining marinade on top of the chicken. Remove pan from the heat and bake in 350 degree oven for 25 to 30 minutes with the bone side down.
SERVES 4

NUTRITIONAL ANALYSIS
Per Portion

Calories	170	Protein	28 gm
Fat	5 gm	Carbohydrate	3 gm
Sodium	77 mg	Cholesterol	68 mg

PORK & BEEF DISHES

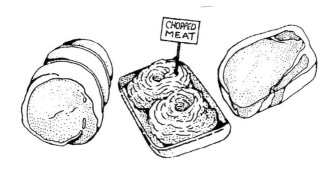

PORK PATTIES
BEEF BOURGUIGNON
BAKED STEAK WITH TOMATO GRAVY
BRAISED BEEF (POT ROAST)
PORK AND BROCCOLI STIR-FRY
FLANK STEAK WITH BURGUNDY SAUCE

Pork Patties

½ Pound Ground Lean Pork
1 Cup Cooked Bulgur Wheat — follow package directions
2 Egg Whites
1 Small Onion — grated
1 Tablespoon Chopped Fresh Parsley (dry will do)
1 Tablespoon Chopped Fresh Mint (dry will do)
   Touch of Black Pepper
1 Small Clove Garlic — minced (optional)
½ teaspoon Vegetable Oil (to oil sheet pan)
   Juice of 2 Lemons

Preheat oven to 350 degrees.
Combine pork and the rest of the ingredients in a large bowl and mix together until well-blended. (Using your hands is the best way.) Form mixture into 6, 3 oz. patties and place on a very lightly oiled sheet pan. Place in a preheated 350 degree oven for 10 minutes. Using a metal spatula carefully turn patties over and cook for an additional 10 minutes. Remove from oven and squeeze lemon juice over the cooked patties. Serve.
YIELDS 6 PATTIES
NOTE: Bulgur wheat is also known as cracked wheat and is available in most grocery stores and health food stores.

NUTRITIONAL ANALYSIS
Per Portion

Calories	99	Protein	10 gm
Fat	3 gm	Carbohydrate	8 gm
Sodium	49 mg	Cholesterol	25 mg

Beef Bourguignon

1 Pound Flank Steak — cut into 1½ inch cubes
1 Medium Onion — peeled and very thinly sliced
½ Tablespoon Vegetable Oil
1 Cup Reduced Sodium Beef Bouillon
½ Cup Red Wine
1 Tablespoon Whole Wheat Flour
   Touch of Black Pepper
¼ teaspoon Oregano

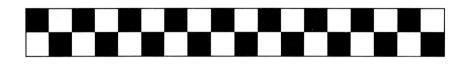

¼ teaspoon Thyme
1 Clove Garlic — minced
1 Pound Fresh Mushrooms — washed and sliced

In an 8-quart dutch oven, saute onions in oil. Add meat and brown on all sides. Pour beef bouillon and red wine in a medium bowl. Add flour, pepper, oregano, thyme and garlic. Stir mixture with a whisk until smooth. Pour over beef and onions mixing thoroughly. Stirring occasionally, simmer for 1 hour. Add mushrooms and continue cooking for another 15 minutes. Add more wine if needed. Serve.
SERVES 4

NUTRITIONAL ANALYSIS
Per Portion

Calories	257	Protein	26 gm
Fat	13 gm	Carbohydrate	10 gm
Sodium	91 mg	Cholesterol	57 mg

Baked Steak with Tomato Gravy

1 Pound Flank Steak — 1 inch thick, with all visible fat removed
  Juice of 2 Lemons
½ teaspoon Vegetable Oil
2 Medium Onions — peeled and sliced
1 Clove Garlic — minced
1 15 oz. Can Stewed Tomatoes (no salt added)
2 teaspoons Brown Sugar
¼ Cup Water
  Touch of Black Pepper

Preheat oven to 350 degrees.
Cut meat into ½ inch thick slices. Sprinkle with lemon juice and let stand for 10 minutes. Put ½ teaspoon oil in a 10″, non-stick skillet over medium to medium-high heat and brown meat. Place in a casserole dish and put onion and garlic on top of meat. Mix brown sugar with stewed tomatoes and pour on top of onions. Pepper to taste. Put cover on dish and bake at 350 degrees for 1 hour.
SERVES 4

NUTRITIONAL ANALYSIS
Per Portion

Calories	257	Protein	24 gm
Fat	11 gm	Carbohydrate	14 gm
Sodium	127 mg	Cholesterol	57 mg

Braised Beef (Pot Roast)

1½ Pounds London Broil or Lean Eye of the Round, all fat removed
½ teaspoon Vegetable Oil
2 Tomatoes — coarsely chopped
1 Onion — chopped
1 Cup Beer
1 teaspoon Italian Spice
1 teaspoon Instant Vegetable Bouillon Granules (low-sodium
  chicken will do)
2 Cloves Garlic — minced
  Touch of Black Pepper
4 Medium Potatoes — cut into wedges (about 1½ pounds)
5 Medium Carrots — cut into 1 inch pieces (about 1¼ pounds)
1 Large Spanish Onion (or 3 medium onions) — cut into ½ inch slices
2 Tablespoons Beer
4 teaspoons Cornstarch

Lightly oil a 12", non-stick skillet and heat over medium-high heat. When skillet is hot, brown beef on all sides. When brown, place beef into an 8-quart dutch oven. Add tomatoes, onion, beer, Italian spice, bouillon granules, garlic and pepper. Bring to a boil, reduce heat, cover and simmer for 1 hour. Add potatoes, carrots and onions, cover and simmer for another 35 to 45 minutes or until vegetables are tender. Using a slotted spoon, transfer meat and vegetables to serving platter. Measure the remaining liquid left in dutch oven. You need 1¼ cups. Mix 2 tablespoons beer and cornstarch together and pour into your dutch oven with 1¼ cups liquid. Stirring constantly with a whisk over medium high heat, cook until mixture is thick. Reduce heat and simmer 1 minute more. Pour sauce over beef and vegetables and serve.
SERVES 6

NUTRITIONAL ANALYSIS
Per Portion

Calories	197	Protein	23 gm
Fat	11 gm	Carbohydrate	1 gm
Sodium	84 mg	Cholesterol	57 mg

Pork and Broccoli Stir-Fry

12 Ounces Lean Pork Loin (all fat removed) —
cut into bite-size thin strips
2 Tablespoons Cornstarch
1 teaspoon Fresh Grated Ginger (dry will do)
1 Tablespoon Reduced Sodium Soy Sauce
1 Tablespoon Sherry
½ Cup Water
½ teaspoon Chicken Bouillon Granules (low-fat, low-sodium)
1 teaspoon Vegetable Oil
8 Green Onions — cut into ¼ inch pieces, green tops, too
6 Cups Broccoli Florets
1 Cup Sliced Water Chestnuts — rinsed and drained

In a small bowl or cup mix together well cornstarch, ginger, soy sauce, sherry, water and bouillon granules. Set aside. Put oil into a 12″, non-stick skillet and place over medium to medium-high heat. When pan is hot, add pork and stir fry for 2 to 4 minutes. Add green onions, cook 30 seconds longer and then add broccoli florets and water chestnuts. Stir fry for 2 minutes more. Add cornstarch mixture and stir in well. Put cover on skillet and cook for 1 to 2 minutes longer. Remove from heat and serve.
SERVES 4

NUTRITIONAL ANALYSIS
Per Portion

Calories	248	Protein	25 gm
Fat	8 gm	Carbohydrate	21 gm
Sodium	256 mg	Cholesterol	51 mg

Flank Steak with Burgundy Sauce

Flank Steak:
1 ¾ Pound Flank Steak — all visible fat removed
1 Cup Burgundy Wine for Marinade
2 Tablespoons Red Wine Vinegar
1 Small Onion — sliced thin

Place steak in glass dish and pour burgundy wine and vinegar on top. Place onion slices on top of steak. Marinate for 2 hours turning once. Remove from marinade and place on a broiler pan. Place under broiler and cook for 4 minutes on each side or to desired doneness. Slice meat very thin (¼ inch) diagonally. Serve with prepared burgundy sauce (directions to follow).

Burgundy Sauce:
1 Cup Burgundy Wine
½ Cup Beef Broth
3 Tablespoons Flour
  Touch of Black Pepper

Place all burgundy sauce ingredients in a small saucepan over high heat whisking constantly. Bring to a boil. When satin smooth and thickened remove from heat and pour over cooked flank steak on serving platter.
SERVES 6

NUTRITIONAL ANALYSIS
Per Portion

Calories	245	Protein	27 gm
Fat	13 gm	Carbohydrate	5 gm
Sodium	100 mg	Cholesterol	66 mg

DESSERTS

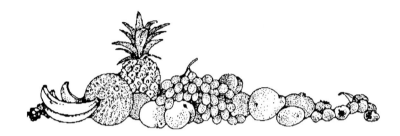

CHOCOLATE SAUCE
STRAWBERRY SAUCE
CREAMY RUM RAISIN SAUCE
CREAMY RICE PUDDING
FRESH FRUIT PLATE WITH
SWEETENED CREAM
FROZEN BANANA
PEACH CRISP
SWEET POTATO CAKE SQUARES

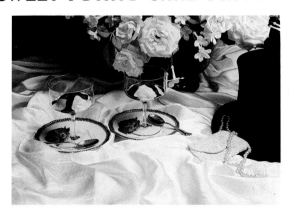

Bananas with
Chocolate Sauce

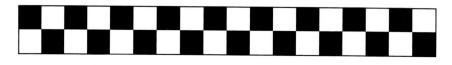

Desserts

I made cheesecake so rich, those who ate it could feel their arteries closing as they dined. Thus I became known as "Captain Cheesecake."

My feelings about dessert run rich and deep (just like my cheesecake), but I know that we're better off without them. However, it doesn't hurt to indulge once in a great while.

While we know that fat makes fat, we also must acknowledge that sugar is sugar is sugar. It doesn't matter whether it's white, brown, liquid, comes from fruit or apple juice concentrate. It's all sugar. If you're not planning on exercising, then plan on not eating sugar because you won't burn it off.

In this next section, you will see that I've created several desserts that are low in calories as well as sugar, and believe me this was no easy task.

Back in my restaurant, The Elegant Pelican, my sweet concoctions were known as the The Grand Finale. These may not quite reach that stature, but they'll certainly do in a pinch when you just want to have something sweet. Enjoy.

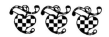

Chocolate Sauce

½ Cup Ricotta Cheese — low-fat, low-sodium
¼ Cup Water
½ Cup Sugar
¼ Cup Unsweetened Cocoa Powder
3 teaspoons Cornstarch
1 teaspoon Vanilla
1 Tablespoon Water or more if needed*

Place ½ cup ricotta cheese in blender with ¼ cup water. Blend until smooth. Pour this mixture into a saucepan and add sugar, cocoa powder and cornstarch. Mix together well with a whisk until smooth. Over medium-high heat, bring to a boil, stirring constantly. Reduce heat and simmer for 30 seconds. Remove from heat and whisk in vanilla and water until smooth.
YIELDS 1 CUP
Look at consistency of chocolate. If it is too thick, add 1 Tablespoon of water at a time and whisk in well.

NUTRITIONAL ANALYSIS
Per 1 Tbsp. Portion

Calories	36	Protein	1 gm
Fat	less than 1 gm	Carbohydrate	8 gm
Sodium	7 mg	Cholesterol	less than 1 mg

Strawberry Sauce

1 10 oz. Package Frozen Strawberries
½ teaspoon Lemon Juice
¼ Cup Sugar

Thaw strawberries and place in food processor bowl with the rest of the ingredients. Blend until smooth.
YIELDS 1¼ CUPS

NUTRITIONAL ANALYSIS
Per 1 Tbsp. Portion

Calories	15	Protein	less than 1 gm
Fat	less than 1 gm	Carbohydrate	4 gm
Sodium	less than 1 mg	Cholesterol	0 mg

Creamy Rum Raisin Sauce

½ Cup Cottage Cheese — low-fat
½ Cup Water
¼-½ Cup Sugar
2½ teaspoons Cornstarch
½ teaspoon Allspice
¼ Cup Raisins
2 teaspoons Rum Extract
1 teaspoon Vanilla

Place cottage cheese and water in blender and blend until smooth. Pour this mixture into a saucepan and add sugar, cornstarch and allspice. Mix together well with a whisk until smooth. Over medium-high heat bring to a boil stirring constantly. Reduce heat and simmer for 30 seconds. Remove from heat and stir in raisins, rum extract and vanilla.
YIELDS 1¼ CUPS

NUTRITIONAL ANALYSIS
Per 1 Tbsp. Portion

Calories	28	Protein	less than 1 gm
Fat	less than 1 gm	Carbohydrate	6 gm
Sodium	23 mg	Cholesterol	less than 1 mg

Creamy Rice Pudding

2 Cups Cooked Rice (follow package directions, but omit salt and butter)
1¾ Cups Skim Milk
¼ Cup Ricotta Cheese — low-fat, low-sodium
⅓ Cup Sugar
1 Tablespoon Vegetable Oil
1 teaspoon Vanilla
  Cinnamon to sprinkle on top

Cook rice according to package directions omitting salt and butter. While rice is cooking, put milk, ricotta cheese, sugar, vegetable oil and vanilla in a blender and process until smooth. When rice is cooked, add milk mixture to rice in saucepan and mix together. Cover and cook for 20 minutes over medium heat stirring often. Remove from heat, spoon into serving dishes and sprinkle cinnamon on top. Serve warm or cold.
SERVES 4

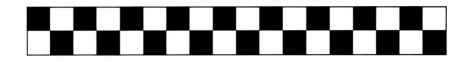

NUTRITIONAL ANALYSIS
Per Portion

Calories	279	Protein	8 gm
Fat	4 gm	Carbohydrate	51 gm
Sodium	72 mg	Cholesterol	3 mg

Fresh Fruit Plate with Sweetened Cream

4 Cups Mixed Fresh Fruit — sliced strawberries, peeled, sliced kiwi
   fruit, fresh sliced peaches, peeled, seeded canteloupe, etc.
2 Tablespoons Tapioca (instant)
1 Cup Water
⅓ Cup Ricotta Cheese — low-fat, low-sodium
3 Tablespoons Sugar
1 teaspoon Vanilla

   Pour 1 cup water in a saucepan and sprinkle in the tapioca. Allow
to sit for 10 minutes. Place saucepan over high heat and bring to a boil
whisking constantly. Reduce heat to low and simmer for 1 to 2 minutes.
Allow this mixture to cool and pour into a blender with ricotta cheese,
sugar and vanilla. Blend on high speed (about 2 minutes) until mixture
is satin smooth. Refrigerate to chill before serving. Portion one cup of fruit
per serving into individual dishes and pour ¼ cup of sweetened cream
over top.
YIELDS 4 FRUIT SERVINGS AND 1¼ CUPS CREAM

NUTRITIONAL ANALYSIS
Per Portion

Calories	140	Protein	4 gm
Fat	1 gm	Carbohydrate	31 gm
Sodium	25 mg	Cholesterol	2 mg

Frozen Banana

4 Ripe Bananas — peeled and cut into ¼ inch slices

Place bananas in plastic bag and put into freezer. When bananas are frozen solid, remove from plastic bag and place them in a food processor. Process until smooth. Scoop into serving dish and pour chocolate sauce on top. Serve immediately.
SERVES 8

NUTRITIONAL ANALYSIS
Per Portion

Calories	52	Protein	less than 1 gm
Fat	less than 1 gm	Carbohydrate	13 gm
Sodium	less than 1 mg	Cholesterol	0 mg

Peach Crisp

2 Pounds Firm Ripe Peaches — peeled and thickly sliced
¼ Cup Light Brown Sugar
½ teaspoon Allspice
  Pinch of Clove
2 Tablespoons Lemon Juice
3 Tablespoons Grape Nuts Cereal

Preheat oven to 375 degrees.
Place all ingredients except Grape Nuts in a medium bowl. Toss together lightly and pour into a 1-quart baking dish. Sprinkle Grape Nuts on top and bake for 45 minutes at 375 degrees.
SERVES 8

NUTRITIONAL ANALYSIS
Per Portion

Calories	74	Protein	less than 1 gm
Fat	less than 1 gm	Carbohydrate	19 gm
Sodium	19 mg	Cholesterol	0 mg

Sweet Potato Cake Squares

Vegetable Non-Stick Cooking Spray
1 16 oz. Can Yams (cut sweet potatoes in syrup) drained
1½ Cups Sugar
¼ Cup Vegetable Oil
2 Cups Flour
2 Eggs
2 Egg Whites
2 Tablespoons Pumpkin Pie Spice
3 Tablespoons Low-Sodium Baking Powder (or 3 Tablespoons of
   regular baking powder)

Preheat oven to 350 degrees.

Spray bottom and sides of a 12"x17" sheet pan with non-stick cooking spray. Place drained sweet potatoes in mixing bowl and mash with a fork. Add the remaining ingredients and beat with an electric mixer on medium to high speed until smooth (about 2 to 3 minutes). Pour sweet potato batter into sheet pan and spread evenly. Bake in preheated 350 degree oven for 20 to 25 minutes. Remove from oven, cool slightly and cut into 3 inch squares.
MAKES 20, 3" SQUARES

NUTRITIONAL ANALYSIS
Per Portion

Calories	158	Protein	2 gm
Fat	4 gm	Carbohydrate	30 gm
Sodium	18 mg	Cholesterol	21 mg

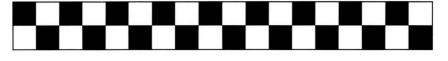

Watch It List

Oil — All types of vegetable oils — remember, fat makes fat

Sugar — Refined white, brown, molasses, honey, corn syrup, barley malt, etc. Sugar is sugar is sugar.

Beverages — Coffee, tea, alcohol, diet soda—especially the ones with caffeine, decaffinated coffee and tea, sugar drinks.

Dairy — Watch out for the words Low-Fat.

Nuts — Pecans, pistachios, walnuts, sunflower seeds, brazil nuts.

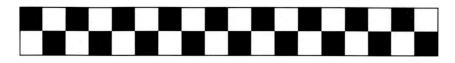

Hold It

Remember these are just guidelines to provide a simple understanding. I'm sure that with a little effort, one could practically write a new dictionary on what not to eat.

Dairy — Cheese, cream cheese, sour cream, heavy cream, half and half, milk, ice cream; all the things we will learn to do without.

Salt — "Lite" salt, table salt, Kosher salt, sea salt, MSG; these are taboo.

Meats — Organ and fatty meats.

Oils — Shortening, mayonnaise, butter, margarine, coconut oil, palm oil, chicken fat, animal fat. Remember—fat makes fat.

Got Anything To Eat?

I know that all this stuff you've read is easier said than done, so here's a help list. These are just a few tips to help get you through the tough times. A small quantity of any food is not going to hurt. When the foods become the bulk of our intake, the problem begins. So here are a few ideas that can help.

Go For It List

Vegetables — Whether fresh or frozen, keep plenty on hand. Try to eat at least four or more, one-cup vegetable servings daily. Include yellow, orange and dark green vegetables.

Fruits — Fresh is best, but frozen or canned are the next best choices. Shoot for eating about three whole fruits daily. (Remember, fruit contains sugar.)

Whole Grains — These include cereals, breads, crackers, whole wheat, pastas, rice, rice cakes, oatmeal. White flour may be used as long as it does not exceed 50 percent of your total grain. Four servings daily are recommended, but be sure they don't exceed 400 calories. Beans, potatoes, yams or any starchy foods should be considered part of the 400 calorie limit.

Fish, Fowl or Lean Red Meats — Fish is the best choice, but chicken is good, too, and better than beef. Cooked scallops, clams and oysters also are acceptable. You should not consume more than four ounces as an absolute maximum for one day.

Legumes — Beans, lentils and peas are about the best bargain nutritionally and at the market. They are high in protein and fiber. Legumes are starchy foods and you shouldn't have more than 400 calories worth a day. Grains and rice should be included in that limit, as well.

Nuts — Chestnuts and canned water chestnuts are the only choices.

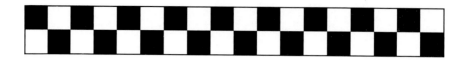

Dairy — Non-fat yogurt, skim milk and non or low-fat cottage cheese and ricotta cheese are all fine. Sap Sago cheese is another option. Two servings of dairy products are recommended per day, but should not exceed 200 calories.

Beverages — Mineral water, vegetable juices, fruit juices (mix fruit juice with seltzer water — ½ fruit and ½ seltzer on ice) herbal teas, hot or cold all offer delicious alternatives to soda pop and other drinks that add calories and contain too much sugar and caffeine. And, of course, don't forget H_2O — 8 glasses daily.